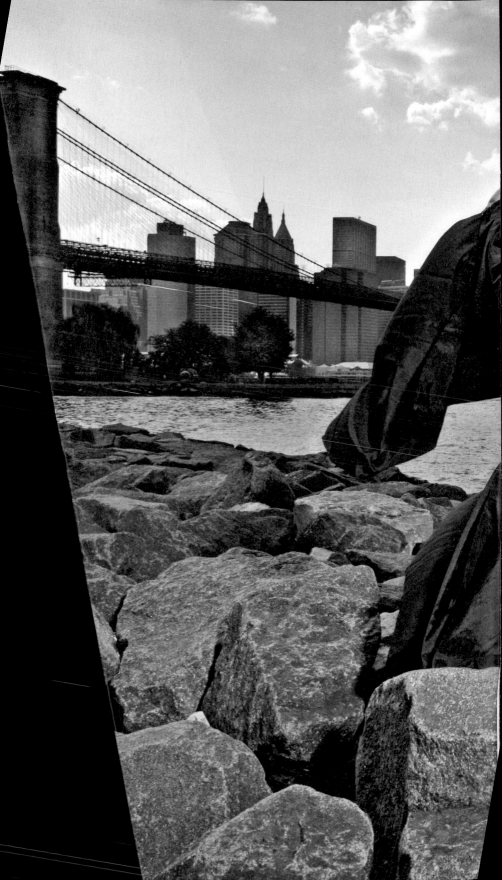

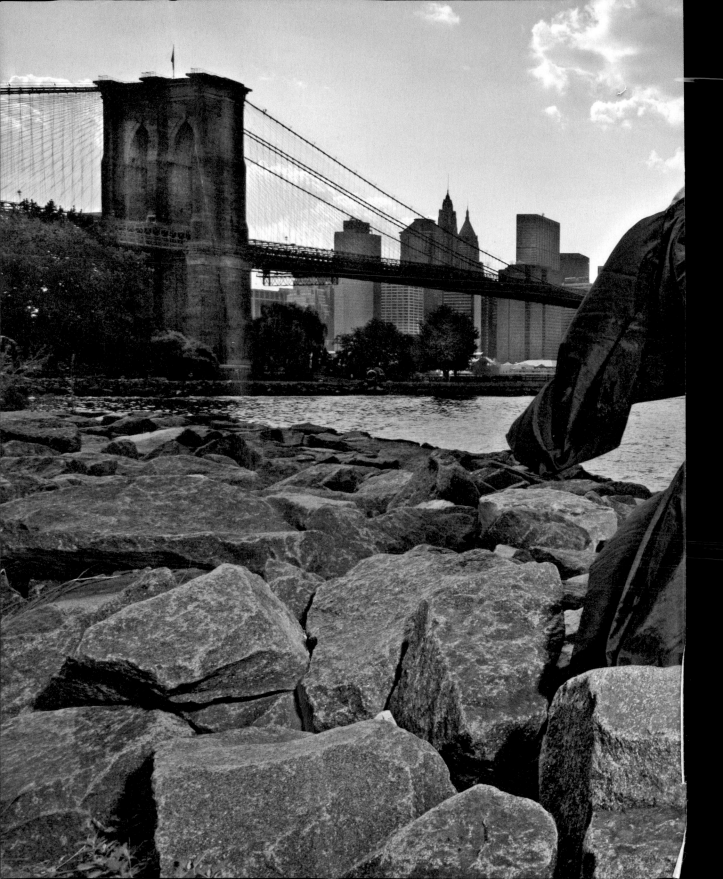

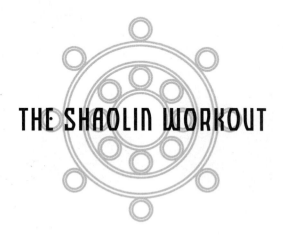

THE SHAOLIN WORKOUT

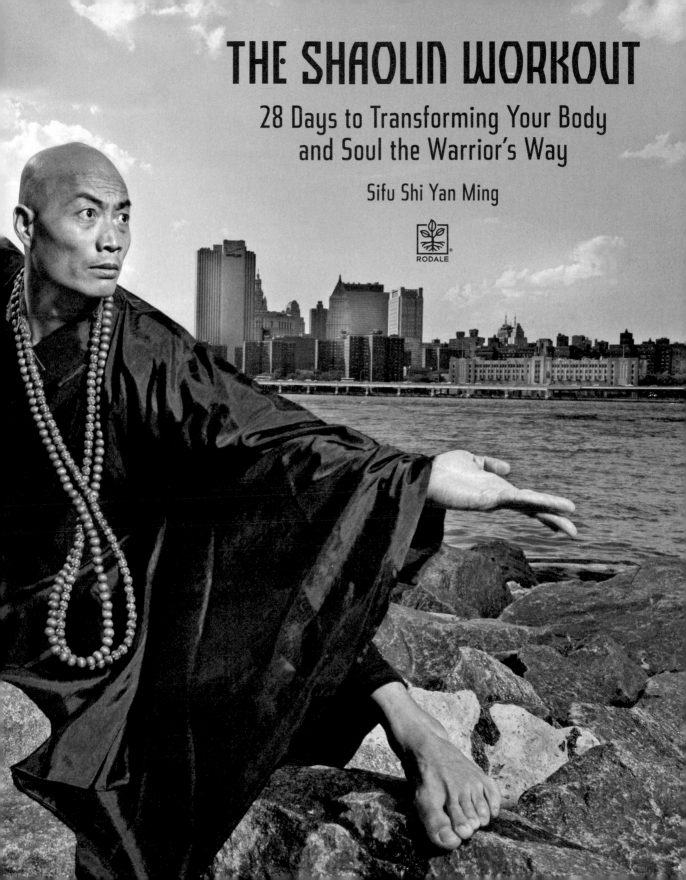

THE SHAOLIN WORKOUT

28 Days to Transforming Your Body and Soul the Warrior's Way

Sifu Shi Yan Ming

RODALE

© 2006 by Sifu Shi Yan Ming

Printed in the United States of America

Rodale Inc. makes every effort to use acid-free ♾, recycled paper ♻.

Photographs by Bob Scott (www.bobscottnyc.com)
Book design by Ellen Nygaard

Library of Congress Cataloging-in-Publication Data

Shi, Yan Ming
    The shaolin workout : 28 days to transforming your body and soul the warrior's way / Sifu Shi
Yan Ming.
        p.   cm.
    Includes index.
    ISBN-13 978–1–59486–400–1   hardcover
    ISBN-10 1–59486–400–4   hardcover
    1. Kung fu—Training.   I. Title.
GV1114.7.S53   2006
613.7′148—dc22   2006003840

Distributed to the trade by Holtzbrinck Publishers

2   4   6   8   10   9   7   5   3   1   hardcover

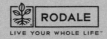

RODALE
LIVE YOUR WHOLE LIFE™

We inspire and enable people to improve their lives and the world around them
For more of our products visit **rodalestore.com** or call 800-848-4735

To my parents, who gave me life
and still watch my every step from above and
whose love I feel at every moment.

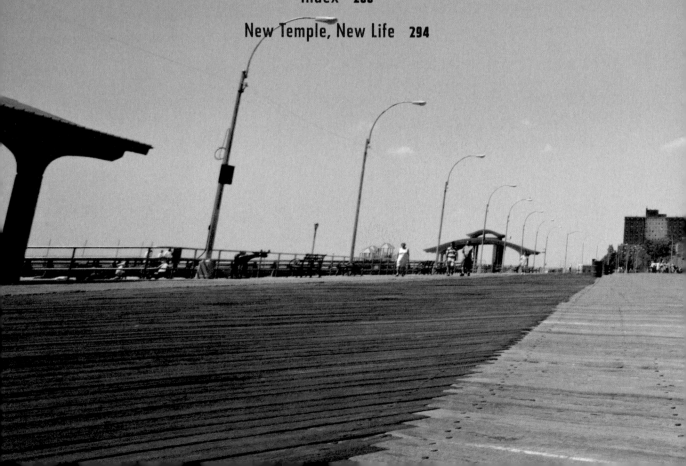

CONTENTS

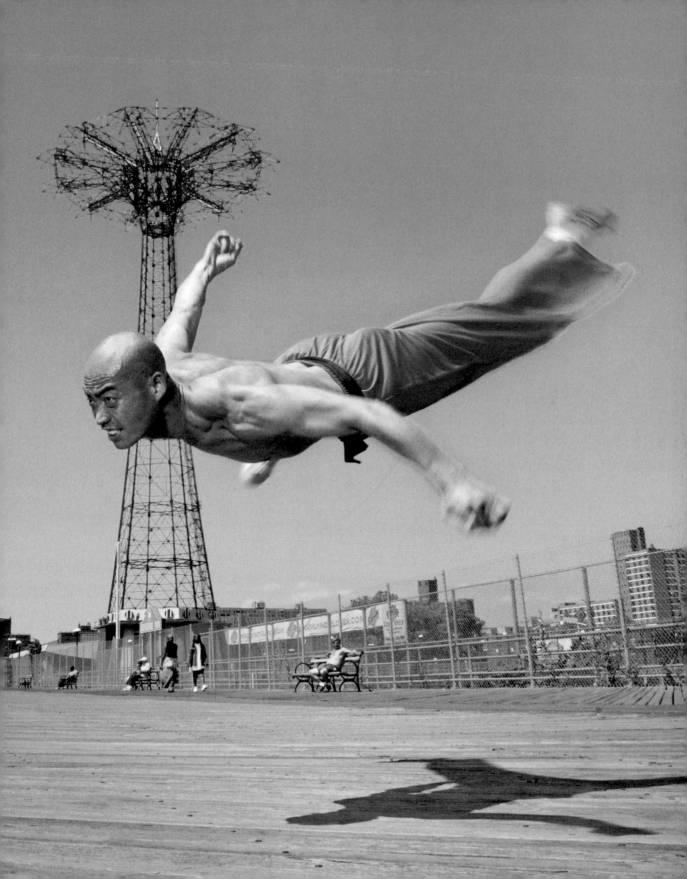

Acknowledgments

This book came together as a result of the efforts of many people, to whom I would like to send thanks:

To Laurie Liss, agent extraordinaire, whose vision this book was from the start, who is my kind of person because she just *does* it. A superb practitioner of action meditation and a great friend as well.

To John Strausbaugh, my coauthor, who worked tirelessly and captured my voice in a way that none other has and who went way, way, way above and beyond the call of duty.

To Sophia Chang, the ultimate partner: in love, in life, in parenthood, in my temple and life journey. The temple would not be what it is without her.

To my remarkable children, Jin Long and Jian Hong, who are my heart and make life even more beautiful 8 days a week, 366 days a year.

To the RZA, my brother in this and many lifetimes, whose support, friendship, and loyalty have helped bring me and the U.S.A. Shaolin Temple to where we are today.

To Zachary Schisgal at Rodale, without whose belief in me this book would not be what it is. To his team, Ellen Nygaard, Andrew Gelman, and Courtney Conroy, whose dedication to this project is evident on every page.

To Heng Ching and Heng Zhong for making me look even more handsome! Thousands and thousands of times over!

To my stellar U.S.A. Shaolin Temple demo team, who always makes me look good.

To Heng Ji, Heng Suo, Heng Nai, Heng Zhi, Heng Xu, Heng De, Heng Fa, Heng Yi, Heng Zhou, Xiao Tian, and everyone else who gave their time and love to read through this book sentence by sentence, word by word.

To the Shaolin Temple in China and all my masters and brothers who helped push me to this place.

To Buddha, for everything.

A special thanks to Jim Jarmusch, John Leguizamo, and the city we call home, New York.

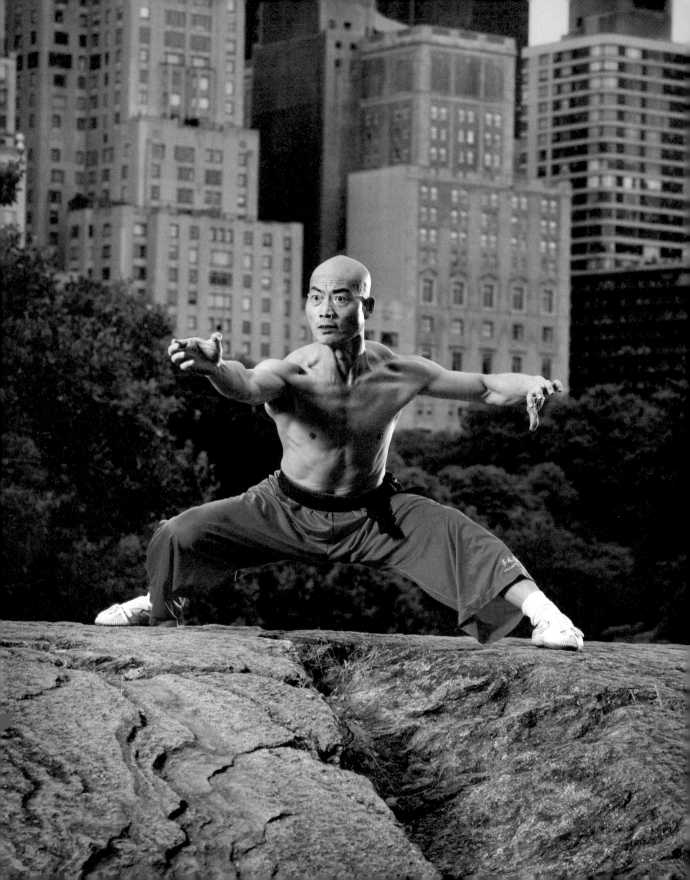

1. Kung Fu, the Way of the Warrior

Before I was born who was I?
After I am born who am I?
Respect yourself, everybody will respect you.
Understand yourself, everybody will understand you.
There are mirrors all around you, strive to see and understand yourself.
Strive to have the heart of a Buddha.
Stop doing bad things, only do good.
Do whatever you can to help others.
In these ways you help yourself.
Help yourself, and you help the world.
Amituofo!

—Sifu Shi Yan Ming

In a typical loft space in Manhattan's hip Greenwich Village, a not-so-typical New Yorker is warming up. He is Sifu Shi Yan Ming, a 34th-generation warrior monk hailing from China's Shaolin Temple, birthplace of Chan Buddhism 1,500 years ago and mecca of all martial arts. Although he is not tall by American standards, his almost impossibly trim body gives an impression of awesome physical power even when he is simply tying the laces of his white training sneakers. With his shaved head and his sternly chiseled good looks, he is the very ideal of the legendary kung fu warrior.

As he begins to move, the impression is more than confirmed. When he stretches his spine, bending forward from the hips and lowering his torso until he can grip his ankles and touch the ground with the top of his head, he makes folding himself in half like a wallet look effortless. Then he executes a series of dazzling kicks, his feet flashing as though he's about to kick a hole in the antique tin ceiling 8 feet above his head. When he punches the air, his fists explode out and back with blinding speed and what one imagines would be devastating force. Then he leaps, and his entire body corkscrews in midair, as though he had ball bearings in place of a lower spine.

It's an amazing display of strength, precision, lightning speed, and incredible agility. He might even go on to break a stack of bricks with his head, slice a stack of boards with his hand, or lean into the points of three spears with his throat—his throat!—and bend the spears rather than be impaled.

1

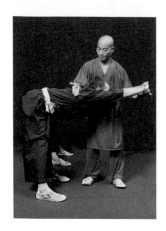

Sifu is a world-renowned master of the martial arts. International action movie stars like Jackie Chan, Chow Yun-Fat, and Michelle Yeoh respectfully address him as "Sifu"—typically translated into English as "Master." So have the thousands of students who have come to this loft space, the U.S.A. Shaolin Temple, to train under him.

A young woman, one of his students, enters the space. Sifu pauses, his body impeccably poised in front of a snarling-dragon mural on the Chinese-red wall. There isn't a dot of perspiration on him. He's not even breathing heavily.

"Amituofo, Sifu!" she calls out.

"Amituofo!" he replies energetically.

Pronounced *ah-mee-toh-foh*, it is the name of one of the three Paradise Buddhas, Amituo ("*fo*" signifies Buddha in Chinese). Saying his name is an international greeting for Buddhists. It is said to show respect, and as a blessing and a prayer. Buddhists chant it as an aid to meditation and often use it as a replacement for common utterances like *hello* and *good-bye, excuse me*, and *thank you*, as a way to stay always mindful of their spiritual lives.

"Merry Christmas!" Sifu then adds—even though it's late spring.

The student smiles. "Happy New Year!" she replies.

It's something else Sifu and his students say often, all year round. Even the letter carrier responds with a laughing "Happy New Year!" when he drops off the day's mail. It's one of Sifu's ways of reminding everyone around him that life is a beautiful gift, and we should celebrate it not just on a few special holidays like Christmas and New Year's, but every day, every hour, every minute—"8 days a week," he likes to say, "and 366 days a year."

More students begin to gather in the space, piling out of the small elevator in

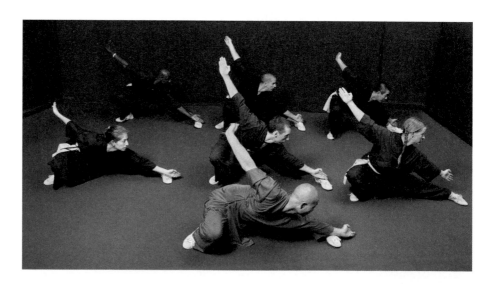

the front, or bounding up the three flights of narrow stairs in the back. The temple lights up with smiles and laughter, with ringing cries of "Amituofo!" and "Happy New Year!" as they hurry into their training uniforms. Twenty, 30, 40 students appear for this particular class.

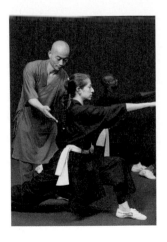

They are male and female, of all sizes, shapes, ages, and ethnicities. They come from all over New York City, from the Bronx to Brooklyn and Queens, or travel in from Long Island and New Jersey. Like Sifu, some of them have come to New York from other countries—Switzerland, India, Germany, Brazil, Korea, Italy, Canada, and Austria, among others. Sifu's students include college students and professors, blue-collar and office workers, movie stars and rap stars, business executives and retail salespeople, yoga instructors, a cop, a doorman, a young Italian apprentice chef, an orchestral composer. Children from as young as 3 to 14 also train at the temple, in their own afternoon classes.

For all their diverse backgrounds, Sifu's students act nothing like strangers who have dragged themselves to the typical gym for a routine class. Everyone greets everyone else by name or nickname, and Sifu knows them all. Everyone is happy and excited to be here. It feels like a large family gathering on a holiday, with Sifu as its patriarch. "He's like a father to us," you often hear students say, even though some of them are older than he is.

"I was amazed at the feeling I had just walking in the door," Sifu's student and disciple Shi Heng Xu recalls of her first time at the U.S.A. Shaolin Temple. "There was this feeling of bliss."

Incredibly, the buzz of high spirits is maintained through the next 2 hours of extremely strenuous training in kung fu, or Chan Quan. (Although "kung fu" is the

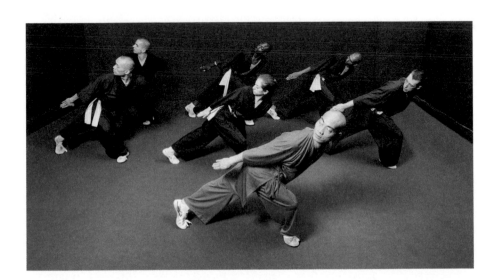

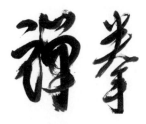

Chan Quan

universally recognized term in the West, Chan Quan—pronounced *chan chwan*—is the proper name for Chan Buddhism or martial arts. In this book we will use "kung fu" and "Chan Quan" interchangeably.) Some of the students in today's class have trained with Sifu for years; some just started today. Some can execute startling leaps and kicks with power and precision; others are just learning. But there is absolutely no sense of competition, showing off, or self-consciousness. In fact, it is just the opposite: Everyone cheers everyone else on, encouraging each student to strive for his or her personal best, which is all Sifu asks of any student.

"Sifu sees everybody's potential," says actor John Leguizamo, who has trained at the temple. "His method is so democratic and fair that way. You only compete with yourself, even though you may see people performing way better than you and way worse than you. It puts your life into perspective in a simple, martial arts kind of way, without words and fancy therapy sessions."

"We all sweat together," Heng Xu explains. "We all go through the pain together. It breaks down your barriers and helps you to be yourself, not just in here but out in the rest of your life."

David, a businessman, makes the 2-hour drive into Manhattan from Long Island three or four times a week to train. In his early forties, he had some 20 years' experience with other exercise and martial arts programs when he first came to the U.S.A. Shaolin Temple.

"I can tell you this is the best workout I've ever had," he says after 8 months of training at the temple. "Nobody ever made me work the way Sifu does." But he stresses that it is far more than just an exercise program. "This is a way to approach your whole life. Sifu has opened my head in all sorts of ways. I've noticed that people who've been coming to the temple for 2, 3 years, or more are all very successful in their lives. I don't just mean that they drive nice cars and have successful careers, although a lot of them do. I mean you can see it in their whole approach to their lives. They respect themselves. People who come to the temple just to get a workout tend not to stick with it. It's as much about the way of living as the physical training. Anybody can show you how to work out. Sifu is about showing you how to live."

Wherever you are, the Shaolin Workout now offers you the same rare opportunity Sifu's New York City students enjoy: the chance to learn the fundamentals of Chan Quan from this Shaolin Temple warrior monk, and the challenge to live the most beautiful life you can. This book is absolutely unique in all the world—just like you are. No book before it, and none that will come after it, is like this book. It is not merely a book of physical exercises, or a book of mental exercises, or a book of spiritual exercises. *The Shaolin Workout* shows you more than a way of training. It introduces you to the warrior's way of life. The second you picked this book up and started to read these words, you began to transform yourself.

The monks of Shaolin Temple have been teaching students Chan Quan for 15 centuries. *The Shaolin Workout* draws on this rich heritage of teaching experience. In this book, Sifu has distilled the fundamentals of kung fu into an introductory course of 28 sessions, which incorporate daily lessons in the mental discipline and spiritual principles that are as essential to Shaolin kung fu as the moves. You will not be a kung fu master when you've successfully completed these sessions. You will not learn how to break boards with your hand. Sifu will teach you the basic stretches, stances, hand strikes, and kicks that are the foundations of this ancient yet living martial art. If you choose to continue learning Chan Quan, you will have a solid base on which to build.

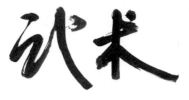

Wu Shu

If you choose to go no further than this program, you will still find yourself transformed, physically, mentally, and spiritually, by your having committed yourself to the program. Sifu will teach you that kung fu is far more than just another exercise program, and it promotes much more than physical health. It is a comprehensive physical, mental, and spiritual discipline. Kung fu is a way of life— a warrior's life of action. Sifu calls it "action meditation." As he guides you through a step-by-step beginner's course in kung fu, Sifu will share his philosophy of life in lessons you can carry throughout your day. If you apply yourself to all aspects of the Shaolin Workout—the mental and spiritual, as well as the physical—you will begin to transform not just your body but your life. You will develop mental clarity and calm, experience an enhanced sense of self-confidence and respect, and learn to appreciate what a beautiful gift your life is every day, every hour, every second.

No one is too young or too old, too weak or heavy, too short or too tall, to train the Shaolin Workout way. You need no prior knowledge of the martial arts or any other training. At the same time, no one is too fit to benefit from training this way, either. No matter what kind of physical training you do now, you will find that the Shaolin Workout enhances your strength, stamina, balance, and grace while improving your mental outlook.

That's true whether you're male or female. Chan Quan is truly gender blind. Women can be as adept at it as men, and often surpass them in speed, flexibility, and grace. Guys know how cool they look when they practice kung fu. And any guy will tell you how great women look when they do it. There is nothing more attractive than a woman who is in great shape and is as confident and poised in her life as she is in her body. Watch any kung fu movie starring Michelle Yeoh or Zhang Ziyi and you'll see for yourself.

The Shaolin Workout does not teach you how to "beat people up." Even though Chan Quan is a warrior's discipline, the vast majority of people who study with Sifu never expect to get into an actual fight on the street. The essence of being a warrior is not looking for people to beat up and dominate. That's just being a bully. Learning kung fu is *not* "learning how to fight," and by teaching it that way, some martial arts instructors make a major error in limiting their students' mental and spiritual understanding. If you want to learn how to beat people up, this workout will be of no use to you. At the U.S.A. Shaolin Temple, Sifu tells new applicants, "If you're looking for a master to teach you how to fight, don't come to me. Go see Yoda."

Yes, Sifu wants you to be able to defend yourself or others in case of an assault, and your Shaolin Workout training will help. But it won't be because you learned some fancy ways to fight. It will be because mastering the Shaolin Workout helps you to be confident in your body and mentally relaxed in moments of crisis or stress so that you can react to an attack with speed and power.

The true way of the warrior is not to seek dominance over others but to achieve mastery of *yourself*. Kung fu helps you do that through training both your body and your mind and promoting mental clarity while it helps you build physical strength, endurance, balance, and flexibility. If you follow this program with dedication, you will find yourself standing taller and straighter, walking more confidently, moving with newfound grace, being less susceptible to aches and pains, and tiring less easily. You will also find that the enormous sense of self-esteem and accomplishment you get from mastering the movements and feeling more physically fit will radiate out through your life, helping you to tackle the world with a warrior's confidence, calm, and poise.

Sifu himself is a living testament to the transformative power of kung fu. Named Gen San by his parents, he was born in 1964 in China's rural Henan Province, not far from Shaolin Temple. He was the seventh of nine children. Seven is, of course, a lucky number. It is also noteworthy that when a highly revered Buddhist monk dies, the other monks build a seven-story pagoda to honor him. Gen San was born not only in the year of the dragon, considered extremely auspicious in Chinese tradition, but on (Chinese) New Year's Day, the luckiest day in the calendar.

At first, though, his life seemed anything but fortunate. His mother and father were both low-level workers in the Communist government. Like everyone else in Henan Province, and most of China, they were desperately poor. Starting in 1958, Chairman Mao's Great Leap Forward—a plan to radically restructure all of China's society and economy from a traditional agrarian base into the world's greatest industrial power— had devastated areas like Henan, uprooting whole communities and making a poor people much, much poorer. Food and medicine were scarce, and many people died.

Three of Sifu's older siblings died of starvation before he was even born. When Sifu himself became ill at the age of 3 and was close to death, his father sold his only possession of any value, a fountain pen, to buy his son medicine. But it didn't help, and when Sifu appeared to have died, the grieving parents wrapped him in blankets and went out on the road from their home, looking for a place to bury him; they could not afford the cost of an official burial place.

On the road, they were met by a man who asked why they were crying. When they said they were on their way to bury their son, he asked if he could take a look at the boy.

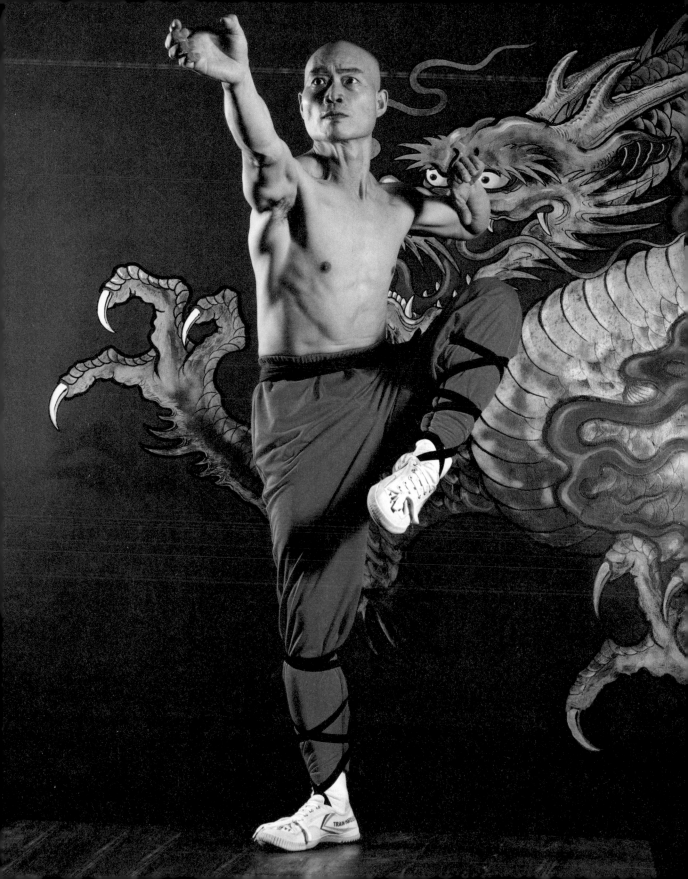

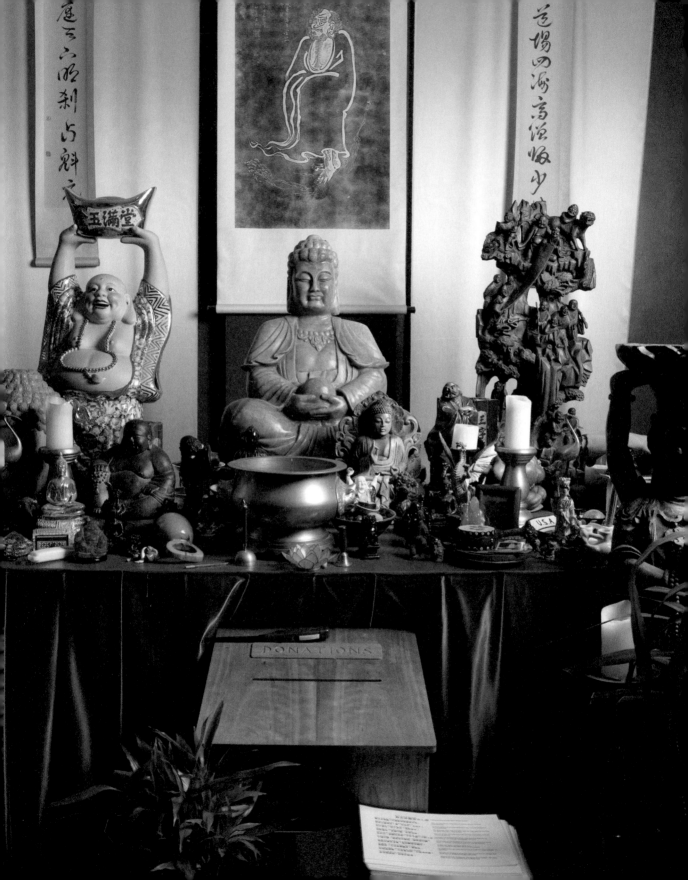

This man, a poor acupuncturist with only a few needles, persuaded them to let him try to save the child. Miraculously, it worked. Sifu has always been convinced that this man was in fact a bodhisattva, a kind of Buddhist saint, sent by Buddha himself. For this reason, he believes it is his duty to repay Buddha's blessing by spreading wisdom and knowledge to as many people in the world as he can. When Sifu was 5, his parents brought him to Shaolin Temple and asked the monks to accept him as a disciple.

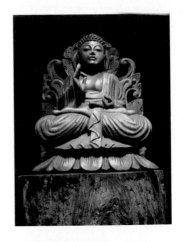

Shaolin Temple was founded in AD 495, but its story really began 2,600 years ago, with the creation of Buddhism in what is now Nepal, a small country between India and China. Buddhism's founder, Siddhartha Guatama (known as Shijiamouni in China), was a Hindu prince who renounced his future kingship and all worldly goods and power. He saw all the suffering in the world and concluded that it was caused by desire. Seeking a way to free the mind and the heart from desire, he meditated for several years and achieved enlightenment, becoming Buddha (Enlightened One). He found the Way, the Dharma.

As Buddhism spread, it developed into many different ways of interpreting and practicing Buddhist principles. Some of these traditions are very caught up in analyzing the voluminous Buddhist writings and observing hundreds of rules: against showing your teeth when you smile, against eating spicy food, against monks looking women in the eye, against looking more than 3 feet around you. In China, this kind of Buddhism is called Xiao Xing— "lesser vehicle" or "small Buddhism"— because it is so narrowly observed and is restricted to just a few adepts.

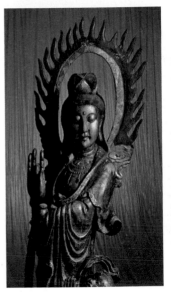

Chan Buddhism, founded at Shaolin Temple, is very different. "Chan" means meditation. Chan is a much simpler form of practice and a more expansive way of life. In Chan, the temple is everywhere; one can pray anywhere and meditate in any position. Chan emphasizes the idea of personal awakening and understanding for everyone, not just a handful of adepts. All things in the universe, Chan Buddhism teaches, are connected by the spiritual life force called chi and are capable of enlightenment. Through meditation and discipline, Chan Buddhists seek to clear their minds and hearts of petty distractions and desires. They believe that if you have an open heart and a pure mind, if you respect and understand yourself, you help spread peace and love in the world.

Shaolin Temple was founded when an Indian monk named Ba Tuo came to China. At that time, China was divided into two kingdoms separated by the Yangtse River. Ba Tuo went to the northern kingdom and asked Emperor Shao Wen for some secluded land where he could found a Buddhist monastery. Ba Tuo went to the Song mountain range in Henan Province and took some land in a forest at the foot of Shao Mountain. In Mandarin, "lin" means forest; the monastery got its name by combining "Shao" and "lin."

Ba Tuo's lineage ended 32 years later. His philosophy of Xiao Xing Buddhism was not continued, because it did not give his followers the correct tools to adapt the philosophy to their needs. However, Ba Tuo did make disciples of two former generals, Hui Guang and Seng Chou. These warriors brought the first martial arts to Shaolin Temple. This was a good thing, because the monastery soon proved to be an irresistible target for local bandits and thieves. Beginning with Hui Guang and Seng Chou, the monks learned how to defend themselves, and thus the tradition of the Shaolin warrior monk was born.

Because Shaolin Temple is revered around the world as the home of martial arts, there is a common misperception that the practice of kung fu began there. In fact, various martial arts were already thousands of years old when the temple was founded. However, it was at Shaolin Temple that they were combined and systematized.

Ba Tuo's successor as abbot of Shaolin Temple also came from India. Bodhidharma, who became known in China as Da Mo, was another prince who renounced his worldly riches and power to pursue a spiritual path.

In AD 527, Da Mo went to a cave on one of the five Breast mountains behind Shaolin Temple, sat down, and began meditating. Da Mo sat facing a wall in the cave and meditated for 9 years. During this time, his disciple Shen Guang (another former general who had renounced that life for the spiritual one) stayed outside Da Mo's cave and acted as a bodyguard for him, ensuring that no harm came to him. Periodically Shen Guang would ask Da Mo to teach him, but Da Mo never responded to Shen Guang's requests. The Shaolin monks would also periodically invite Da Mo to come down to the temple, where he would be much more comfortable, but he never responded.

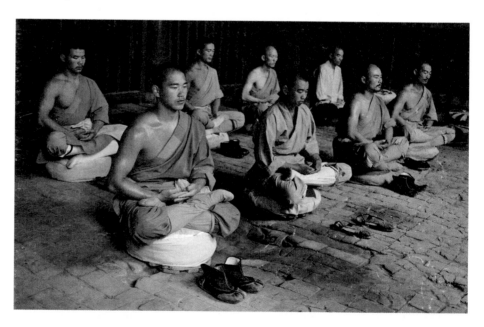

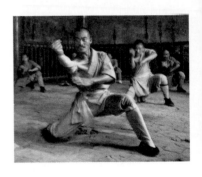

Toward the end of the 9 years, the Shaolin monks built a special room for him. They called this room the Da Mo Ting. When this room was completed, the Shaolin monks again invited Da Mo to come stay there. Da Mo simply stood up, walked down to the room, sat down, and immediately began meditating. Shen Guang stood guard outside his room. Da Mo meditated for another 4 years. Shen Guang would occasionally ask Da Mo to teach him, but Da Mo continued meditating.

By the end of this 4-year period, Shen Guang had been following Da Mo for 13 years, but Da Mo had never said anything to him. It was winter, and Shen Guang was standing in the snow outside the window to Da Mo's room. Cold and angry, he picked up a large block of snow and ice and hurled it inside. The snow and ice made a loud noise as it broke in Da Mo's room, waking Da Mo from his meditation. He looked at Shen Guang. In anger and frustration, Shen Guang demanded to know when Da Mo would teach him.

Da Mo responded that he would teach Shen Guang when red snow fell from the sky. As Shen Guang heard this, something inside his heart changed, and he took the sword he carried from his belt and cut off his left arm. He held the severed arm above his head and whirled it around. The blood from the arm froze in the cold air and fell like red snow. Seeing this, Da Mo agreed to teach Shen Guang. To pay respect for the sacrifice Shen Guang made, disciples and monks of the Shaolin Temple still greet one another using only their right hand, and the name Da Mo Ting was changed to Li Xue Ting—"Li Xue" means "Standing in Snow."

It was Da Mo who founded Chan Buddhism as the abbot of Shaolin. Da Mo also encouraged the development of Chan Quan. In fact, Sifu stresses that there is no separation between the spiritual principles of Chan Buddhism and the physical training of Chan Quan; they are one and the same, totally integrated as action meditation. To emphasize this, Sifu says not "Chan Buddhism *and* martial arts" but always "Chan Buddhism *or* martial arts." There is no difference.

When he became abbot, Da Mo saw that the monks were stiff and out of shape from too much time meditating or bent over religious texts. He understood that a healthy mind needs a healthy body to live in; as Sifu says, "Stretch your body, and you stretch your mind." Under Da Mo and his successors, Shaolin monks became the world's experts in kung fu. They used the skills they developed to defend the monastery, to promote health, and as a form of spiritual and physical discipline.

For 35 generations now (Sifu represents the 34th), Shaolin monks have preserved, developed, and perfected Da Mo's comprehensive system of physical training and spiritual development that transforms the body and mind into an integrated unit. Within the larger system of Chan Quan movements, there are numerous specific styles, some focusing on particular areas of the body (such as Iron Head, Iron Leg, Iron Fist) and many based on close observation of the defensive and offensive tactics of other creatures. Da Mo developed five animal forms:

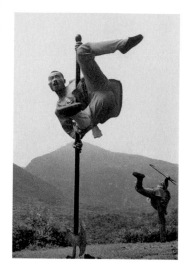

Dragon, Tiger, Leopard, Crane, and Snake. The warrior monks became renowned as excellent horsemen and as masters of the Shaolin Chan Quan art of deploying an array of hand weaponry. It's a good thing Buddhists believe in reincarnation, because it would truly take more than a lifetime to master all of the techniques and skills that come under the general term *kung fu*.

Over the centuries, emperors often enlisted Shaolin warrior monks to help them defend their thrones against upstart warlords or invaders from Japan and Manchuria. One emperor, Emperor Li of the Tang Dynasty, was so grateful to 13 Shaolin warrior monks who saved his life that he released all Shaolin Temple monks from their vows of abstaining from alcohol and eating meat. Emperors frequently rewarded the monks with gifts of money and land, and the temple's estate grew large and prosperous—and all the more attractive to bandits. Shaolin Temple monks are also the only sect of Buddhist monks in the world allowed to practice kung fu.

Yet very often the same emperors who employed the monks and rewarded their services also mistrusted and feared their power. The long history of Shaolin Temple is marked by much betrayal and repression. Shaolin Temple has been attacked, burned, reduced to rubble, and rebuilt a number of times. In the 1600s, Manchu invaders gradually took control of China away from the last emperors of the Ming

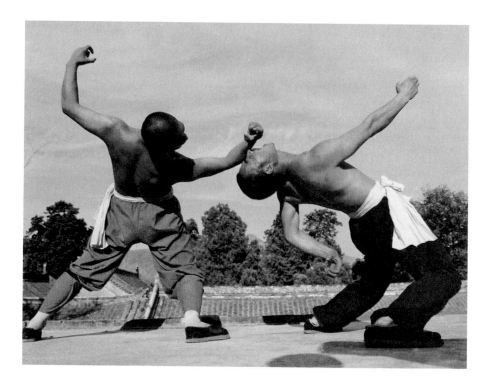

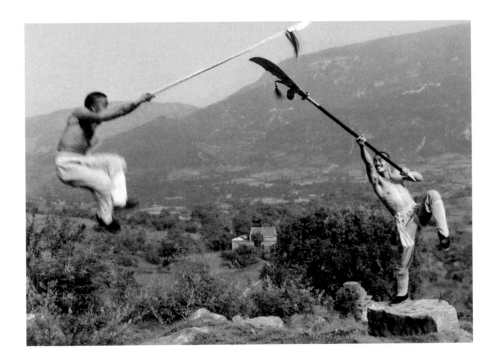

Dynasty. They besieged and destroyed Shaolin Temple, many monks were killed, and the practice of Shaolin kung fu was outlawed. Though much knowledge was lost, the tradition was kept alive in secret.

Feuding warlords destroyed much of the monastery again in 1928. It is said that the temple and surrounding woods burned for more than 45 days. When Mao Zedong established a Communist government, it sought finally to eradicate all religions in China—including Buddhism, as well as Shaolin and the kung fu tradition. Many monks and nuns were executed, others were "reeducated," and practicing kung fu became a crime punishable by death. Ironically, at the same time that he was trying to destroy the temple, Mao employed a Shaolin monk as his personal bodyguard. At the height of Mao's Cultural Revolution, from the mid-1960s to the mid-1970s, the Red Guard stormed Shaolin Temple. Through much of the 20th century, kung fu was better known and appreciated outside of mainland China than in its birthplace.

Despite all the many times that the actual buildings and lands of Shaolin Temple have been attacked, destroyed, rebuilt, and attacked again, the philosophy and traditions remained strong and intact, passed down from one generation of monks to the next, and spread throughout China and the world by traveling monks and their disciples. As the monks have often informed those who threatened to tear down the temple, the building itself is only bricks and wood. The real Shaolin Temple lives in the hearts and minds of each and every monk and disciple and can never be destroyed. That's how Sifu was able to bring Shaolin with him to the United States, and found a new temple in the heart—and hearts—of New York City.

And now he brings it to you. Because the temple is everywhere.

When Sifu entered the Shaolin monastery at the age of 5, it was a particularly low period in its history. Outlawed and suppressed by Mao's government, harassed by the youthful zealots of the Red Guard, the temple had lost all of its land and power, and the monks were reduced to a handful of mostly older men. As one of the few youths, Sifu was doted on and received a great deal of attention.

This did not translate into a soft life. In the Shaolin tradition, the boy was rigorously disciplined and trained, developing the full integration of the physical, mental, and spiritual discipline that is the essence of Chan Buddhism, or Chan Quan. He devoted innumerable hours to action meditation. He chopped wood with his bare hands. He learned to sleep standing on one foot. He endured suspending a 50-pound weight from his testicles, an exercise called "Iron Egg," which toughens the groin until it can withstand a direct kick. He learned to break bricks with his head, hand, or elbow with no pain. He developed the muscles of his neck so that he could lean directly into the blades of spears and bend the spears without pain or injury to the neck.

As a young man, he was honored as both a monk and a master of the martial arts. His full name and titles that were given to him at Shaolin Temple—Sifu Shi Yan Ming— acknowledge this. "Sifu" is translated as "Master"; it also means "Teacher" ("Si") and "Father" ("Fu"). It is the honorific by which his students and admirers always address him. Shi—that's the way it's spelled in English, though it is pronounced more like *shir*, like "sir" with an *h*—is based on the Chinese name of Buddha, Shijiamouni, and denotes that he is a follower of Buddha and a monk. Yan signifies that he represents the 34th generation of Shaolin Temple monks, a continuous lineage going back to the Sung Dynasty. Ming is the name his Sifu gave him; it means "sun and moon," "night and day."

Beginning in the 1970s, kung fu movies from Hong Kong and Taiwan became hugely popular around the world, making international stars of actors such as Bruce Lee, Jackie Chan, Jet Li, and Michelle Yeoh. Many of these films focused on the history and legends of Shaolin Temple and its warrior monks. Sifu was a teenage monk when Jet Li came to the monastery in 1980 to film *The Shaolin Temple*, a unique collaboration between the Communist government and the Hong Kong film industry.

Shaolin Temple has enjoyed one of its periodic renaissances ever since. The teaching and demonstration of martial arts became a flourishing industry in Henan Province. Shaolin Temple, refurbished to its historic glory (it's been jokingly called the Colonial Williamsburg of martial arts), attracts more than a million visitors a year. More than 60 secular martial arts schools in the area attract tens of

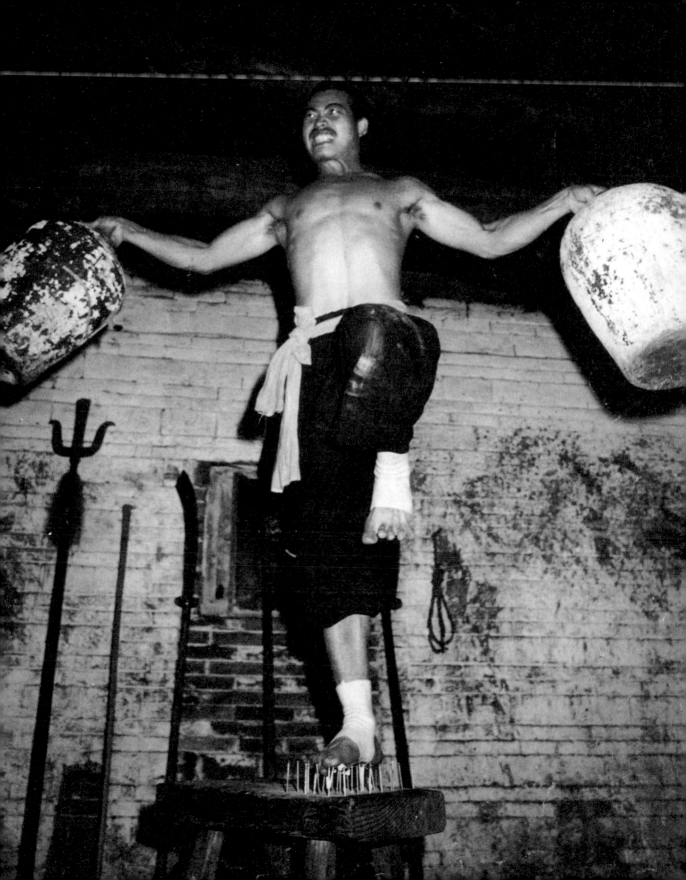

thousands of students from throughout China and from around the world. Some hope to become the next Jet Li. Others practice the martial arts for the spiritual, mental, and physical discipline. There are thousands of kung fu schools around the world, honoring and representing (some more accurately than others) the teachings and traditions that began at Shaolin Temple over 1,500 years ago. In 2004, roughly 7 million people in the United States alone were studying and practicing kung fu.

As a young monk living at Shaolin Temple through the 1980s, Sifu met many visitors from outside China, and he became more convinced than ever that it was his destiny to help spread the Dharma to the rest of the world. In 1992, for the first time in history, a troupe called the Shaolin Temple Fighting Monks came to the United States for a nationwide tour, beginning in Seattle and visiting Boston, New York, and many other cities before its final stop in San Francisco. Its performances showcased the amazing skills of the monastery's finest kung fu practitioners—and Sifu was the undisputed star. With his chiseled good looks and fantastically toned body, he seemed the very ideal of the kung fu warrior. He moved with lightning speed, dazzling grace, and awesome power. And he was a natural showman . . . or, as *Time* magazine genially noted, "a born ham."

Sifu had come to the United States with a private plan. Around midnight after the last performance of the tour, in the San Francisco hotel where the troupe was staying, he approached the handful of official chaperones and watchdogs the Chinese government had sent along with the monks. He said he was just stepping out to take a few snapshots of San Francisco as mementos. Little did they know he was about to become their worst nightmare. He walked out of the hotel and straight into a taxi. Speaking not a single word of English, he simply pointed straight ahead.

The driver pulled away. Knowing nothing of San Francisco, Sifu continued to direct the driver by pointing—go forward, turn left, turn right. He chose streets at random, simply trying to get as far away from the hotel as possible. Today he wryly notes that he was using "action language," just as he does when demonstrating forms to his kung fu students. When the driver realized his passenger had no idea where they were heading, he pulled over and flagged down a passing police car. Sifu showed the officers a copy of his passport, and a collection of newspapers he'd gathered during the tour, with articles about it that featured photographs of him. The cops scratched their heads and instructed the driver to take him somewhere people spoke Chinese.

So the cabbie drove him to a Chinese restaurant. Sifu remembers how excited he was to see the Chinese sign. It was well after midnight and the restaurant was closed, but the staff recognized the star of the Shaolin show and opened up. They spoke Cantonese and could not understand his Mandarin, but they communicated in writing (most of the characters are the same in both). He told them he wanted to defect to the United States and gave them the telephone number of a contact person—a friend of a friend—living in San Francisco.

It's noteworthy that Sifu waited until the entire tour had been completed before he acted on his plan. He could far more easily have defected when the tour went to New York City, the place that was his ultimate goal. But to him, that would have been dishonorable and dishonest. He had committed to performing in the tour, and he could not abandon that responsibility. He determined to finish the tour, completing his commitment to his fellow monks, before acting on his own behalf.

Sifu hid in his new friend's basement for a week, watching the news on TV announcing that the star of the Shaolin troupe had gone "missing" while the frantic chaperones back at the hotel foresaw their grim reception in Beijing when they returned without him. The friend then took him to the airport and put him on a flight to New York, where another contact was waiting to greet him. New York City had always been Sifu's goal. He believed it to be the capital and crossroads of the world, where he could reach out to the most people.

In Manhattan, he hid for 6 months in an apartment above a Buddhist temple in Chinatown. At one point, representatives of the Chinese consulate appeared at his door and tried to convince him to return to China. He politely declined. He also declined to seek political asylum in the United States. He had not left China for political reasons, but to pursue his global mission. U.S. immigration officials were only too happy to provide him with a green card—though they pondered registering his hands as lethal weapons.

In 1994, Sifu opened his first U.S.A. Shaolin Temple over a grocery store in Chinatown, with fewer than 10 students at the start. The space was so small and the ceilings so low that they could barely practice. There was no electricity, so for lighting they fastened flashlights to the walls. Sifu ate and slept in the space. Eventually, he was able to move to a somewhat larger space on the Bowery, a part of Lower Manhattan previously known for its dive bars and flophouses, and then to the current temple in the East Village. Occupying the third floor over a jeans store, the newest incarnation of the U.S.A. Shaolin Temple is reached by what more than one of his students have good-naturedly dubbed "the slowest elevator in Manhattan." Sifu himself jokes that it is the "first chamber" of the temple. Many students prefer to bound up the three flights of narrow stairs, displaying the joyful and apparently limitless energy that characterizes those whose lives have been changed by Sifu's guidance.

With its long, carpeted floor, its floor-to-ceiling mirrors, and closet-size changing rooms, the space is similar to many dance-rehearsal spaces and yoga studios in Manhattan. But as you step out of the elevator to face that dragon mural and a large altar crowded with Buddhas, bodhisattvas, and gently smoking incense, you instantly recognize that this is no ordinary space. Even when the room is filled with a class of students leaping through the air and kicking toward the ceiling, there is a sense of respectful calm, peaceful joy, and highly disciplined order.

In New York City, Sifu is a living example of the Chan Buddhist's principle of

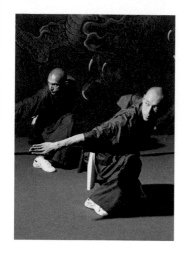

adapting to one's cultural surroundings to better spread peace, love, and knowledge. He realized early on that to help spread the martial arts tradition in the West, he needed to make both himself and his practice approachable. So one is just as apt to see him in sneakers and a U.S.A. Shaolin Temple T-shirt as his yellow and orange monk's robes. Even in this casual "camouflage," you can spot him three blocks away by his walk: Head and chin up, shoulders back, back erect, chest open, he strides quickly along Broadway's crowded sidewalks, with the confident gait of a man who approaches the world openly, or as he puts it, "eye to eye and heart to heart." He drinks beer and champagne, which he calls "special water" and "very special water," eats beef ("American bean curd"), and is a proud and happy father. He likes hip-hop music, and peppers his speech with funky slang like, "Yo, yo, yo! Peace love! Represent! Aiight?" He is, as one of his students told *Time* magazine, "mad cool."

Sifu clearly enjoys life immensely, likes to laugh and kid around, is gentle and sweet with his children. All of this is perfectly in keeping with Shaolin tradition. Since Da Mo's time, the Shaolin monks have rarely conformed to stereotyped images of Buddhist monks living in silent isolation from the world. Shaolin has always evolved with the times. It remains relevant in our 21st-century world, because the true essence of Shaolin is to be flexible in body and mind. Shaolin monks have always spread the Way just as Sifu does, by going out into the world and engaging with people as they live their lives. Wherever he is, with whomever, Sifu is always fully present, in the moment, relaxed and focused.

Sifu uses the traditional Chinese word for a Buddhist monk, He Shang (pronounced *huh shang*), to illustrate the true role of a Chan Buddhist monk in the world. As written in Chinese characters (和尚), it is a fusion of three words into one with a very special meaning. By itself, the first character on the left, *He*, means

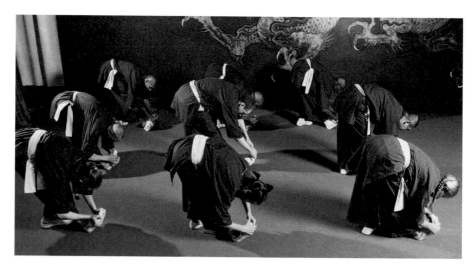

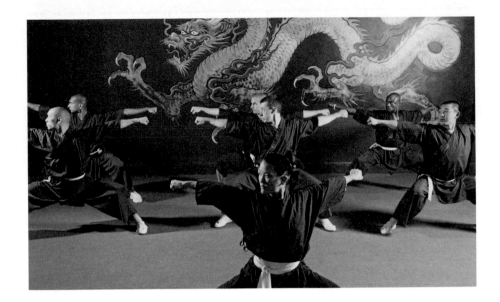

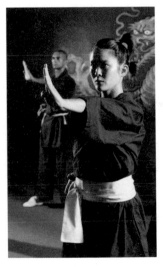

"a living tree." The boxlike character in the middle, *Qu*, means "mouth." The third character, *Shang*, means "intelligence" or "knowledge."

Put together in "He Shang," they mean a person who lives in kind and beautiful harmony with all other things and creatures in the universe; a person who has true knowledge of himself and the universe and speaks that knowledge to others, spreading understanding, peace, and love. It's the monk's understanding and his relationships with everything in the world that make him a monk, Sifu explains, not the shaved head, orange robes, or the monastery with its hundreds of rules.

"Not everyone who shaves his head is a monk," Sifu explains. "And not every monk shaves his head. Every monk does not live in a monastery, and not everyone living in a monastery is a monk. You might see 500 people with shaved heads in a monastery, and maybe none of them is a monk. You may see a man living on the street like a homeless person. He may be a monk. Everywhere can be the temple, and the temple is everywhere. The temple is in your heart. That's why you don't have to go to China to study Chan Buddhism or the martial arts. You can study in New York City, or in your home, anywhere."

When training or teaching, Sifu is an imposing master, supremely disciplined, his attention focused and as razor sharp as the edge of a sword. He is as demanding of his students as he is of himself, encouraging them with shouts of "More chi! Train harder!" Students quickly learn to follow Sifu's few, simple rules of conduct, designed to promote a respectful, clean, and dedicated atmosphere. The students understand and accept the key role discipline plays in their training. It isn't a boot camp, and no one obeys the rules out of intimidation. They do it out of the love and

(continued on page 22)

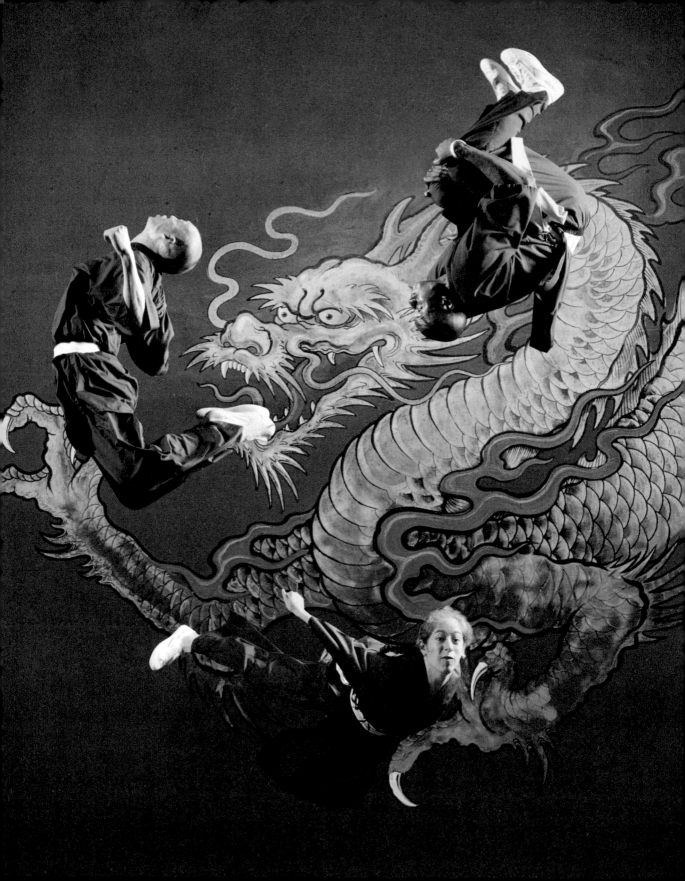

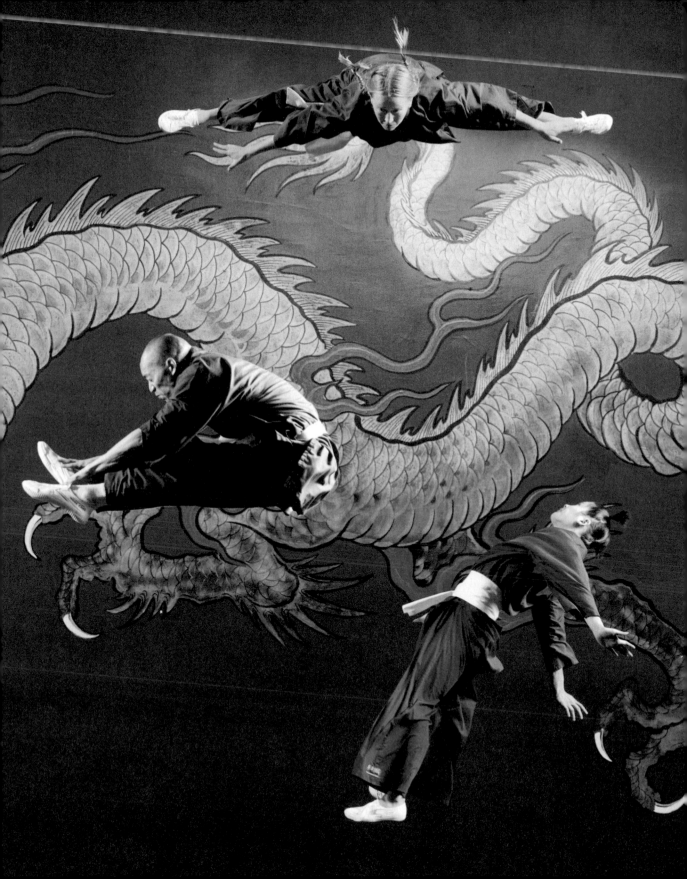

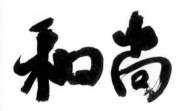

He Shang

enormous respect they have for Sifu, for one another, for themselves, and for the Shaolin tradition. They do it for the positive results they see in their entire lives.

In the Shaolin Workout, Sifu is equally demanding of you. You will quickly find that he is simply challenging you to challenge yourself—to do the best you can today, and do a little better tomorrow, polishing your body, your mind, and your life every day.

It's very important to understand that these two modes, the playful and the serious, are not contradictions or "opposite sides of one coin." They are in complete harmony. Sifu teaches you that it is through the serious training that you develop the physical and mental lightness to fully appreciate the beautiful gift that is your life. The discipline leads to the joy, and the joy in turn leads to the discipline. As you progress in the Shaolin Workout, you will begin to experience the truth and wisdom of this way of life. It's easy to be brave and happy when everything's going well. When you develop a relaxed mind in a relaxed body, when you have self-respect and self-confidence, you see your whole life, the "good" days and the "bad," in a positive light. This is the warrior's way.

"Keep your life simple," Sifu often reminds his students. One minute he's standing in hot video lights, being interviewed for a television program. The next he's down on his hands and knees with a child's scissors in his hand, looking for stray threads in the training area's carpet with the same focus he brings to kung fu. Although he works with many movie stars and pop stars, he's at the U.S.A. Shaolin Temple every day—8 days a week, 366 days a year—teaching his regular students. He leads both beginner and advanced classes in kung fu, as well as courses in tai chi and chi kung (similar to yoga, but more active and fluid). After a strenuous 2-hour kung fu class, Sifu will often share a meal of Vietnamese takeout with students (the restaurant is across the street from his original temple in Chinatown). They sit cross-legged on the ground together, laughing in casual conversation, often with an action movie (Bruce Lee one afternoon, Vin Diesel the next) or some anime for the kids playing on the TV in the corner.

"Yan Ming (is) more down-to-earth than tree roots," the *International Examiner* once declared, and "supremely chill."

Every day after school, children from tots to teens come to the temple to train. Sifu is especially devoted to what he calls "the babies." Many a parent might be very pleasantly shocked to see tiny kids so happy to learn, and so focused and attentive. Some are the children of parents who were already training at the temple. And sometimes it's the other way around. For instance, young mother Heng Ji first saw the temple when she enrolled her 3 1/2-year-old son.

"I loved the changes I saw in him right away," she recalls. "He's much more focused. He follows through." She soon became a student herself, and a devoted disciple.

Like Heng Ji, some of Sifu's students have chosen to take their devotion to Shaolin and to their sifu to a higher level: Just as he was a disciple to his sifu, they have become disciples of Sifu Shi Yan Ming, dedicating themselves to the U.S.A. Shaolin Temple and

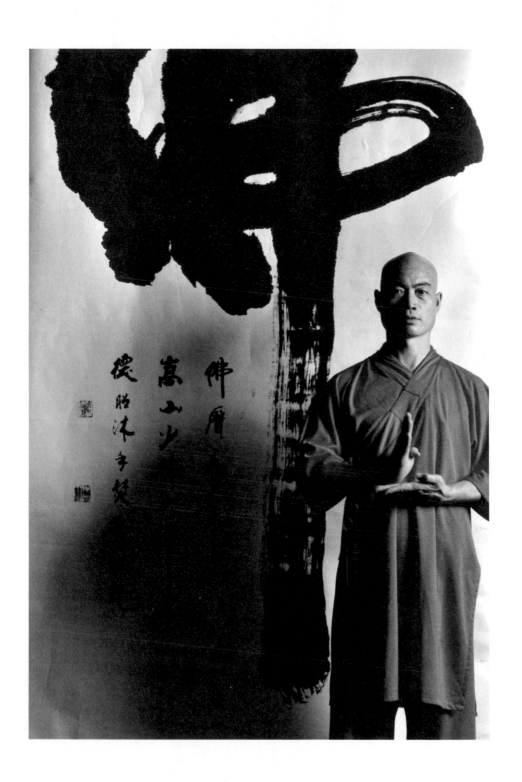

to its traditions of kung fu, or Chan Buddhism. To symbolize their new lives, they are given Chinese names, all beginning with "Heng" (pronounced *huhng*), which follows the same Shaolin tradition by which Sifu's master named him. It signifies that they represent the 35th generation of Shaolin, just as Sifu represents the 34th.

Many of them, male and female, shave their heads like Sifu's to symbolize this new phase of their lives. If you ever meet a fit-looking non-Asian man or woman with a shaved head who goes by a name like Heng Fa or Heng Po, don't be surprised. Sifu says that shaving their heads is one way to simplify their lives. When they get up in the morning and wash their faces, they can wash their heads at the same time! They don't have to think about shampooing, drying, and fixing their hair. It is also quite functional and comfortable when doing rigorous kung fu workouts.

But Sifu emphasizes that it's not required. It would be most unlike Chan Buddhism to have a rule that monks or disciples must cut their hair. You can be a monk or disciple and grow your hair down to your waist, if that's how you honestly express your life. The goal of Chan Buddhism is to be yourself and express yourself fully, not to follow arbitrary rules.

"I come here as a corrective," Heng Ji explains. "I work in an investment bank, and the culture there is so stressful. You work 36 hours straight sometimes. There's a gym in the building, and I often say the people there can't see the ground, much less touch it. These are people in their thirties, and they're on blood pressure medicine. The only exercise some of them get is the annual stress test on the treadmill."

Heng Ji had always worked out and taken yoga and Thai boxing classes. "But I never had the kind of experience I've had at the temple. It's completely different

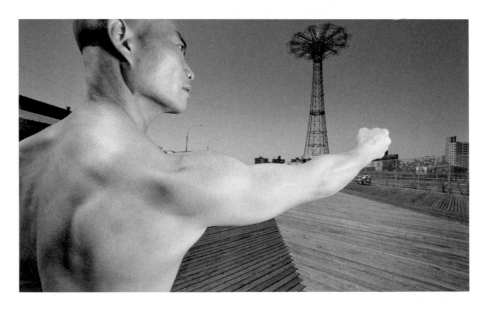

here. You train your body, your mind, *yourself*. I'm much more focused and relaxed now. I put the focus on what's important. At work, not everything is an emergency anymore. I don't obsess about every little thing, which is the culture of the job. I'm hooked." She smiles. "I come here to train 6 days a week."

Heng Li is in his early twenties. After just a few months of training, his friends could see definite changes in him. He laughs, recalling one friend who asked him, "'Why are you walking that way? You walk like you own the city.' I realized I was walking like Sifu does—you stand up straight and face the world. It affects your whole attitude about yourself and life."

Shi Heng Xu had just moved to Manhattan and taken a job in a nearby store when she first visited the temple, 6 years ago. She had been working out at a gym and taking some martial arts classes, but let her gym membership lapse after her first few lessons with Sifu.

"This is just very different," she says. "My other martial arts training was all self-defense and contact fighting. Here, it's more an art form, with a much stronger emphasis on the philosophy."

Like many others—and as you will find, too—her training with Sifu changed her whole life for the better.

"I always wanted to be a more positive person, and now I am," she says. "I changed as a person. I notice that when I'm not able to train, I get moody and grouchy. My boyfriend says, 'Go to kung fu—please!' I don't get angry or frustrated so easily. Training this way, you really learn how to 'flatten your heart,' as Sifu says. After training so hard, what you might encounter out in the world becomes easier to deal with. Mastering your body and your mind gives you the confidence to handle things that come up in your life."

Sifu has continued to be a star in America. Early on, he met Sophia Chang, his soon-to-be life partner. Sophia was the manager of the now-deceased rapper ODB, member of the Staten Island–based hip-hop group the Wu-Tang Clan. Like many hip-hop artists, the Wu-Tang were ardent and longtime fans of kung fu films. Their group's name was inspired by the 1981 kung fu movie *Shaolin and Wu-Tang*. They incorporated their understanding of Shaolin philosophy into their own thinking and codes of conduct, and they even renamed Staten Island "Shaolin."

Sophia introduced them to Sifu in 1995, and they formed a lasting bond of friendship and mutual respect. Wu-Tang's leader and "abbot," the RZA (pronounced *rizza*), became Sifu's first American disciple. "When Sifu came to us, I think destiny brought it to us," RZA writes in his book *The Wu-Tang Manual*. "Then we had a living example of the actual principles. I learned that kung fu was less a fighting style and more about the cultivation of the spirit." He told the magazine *Kungfu*, "I value most the harmony that it can bring to your mind and your body."

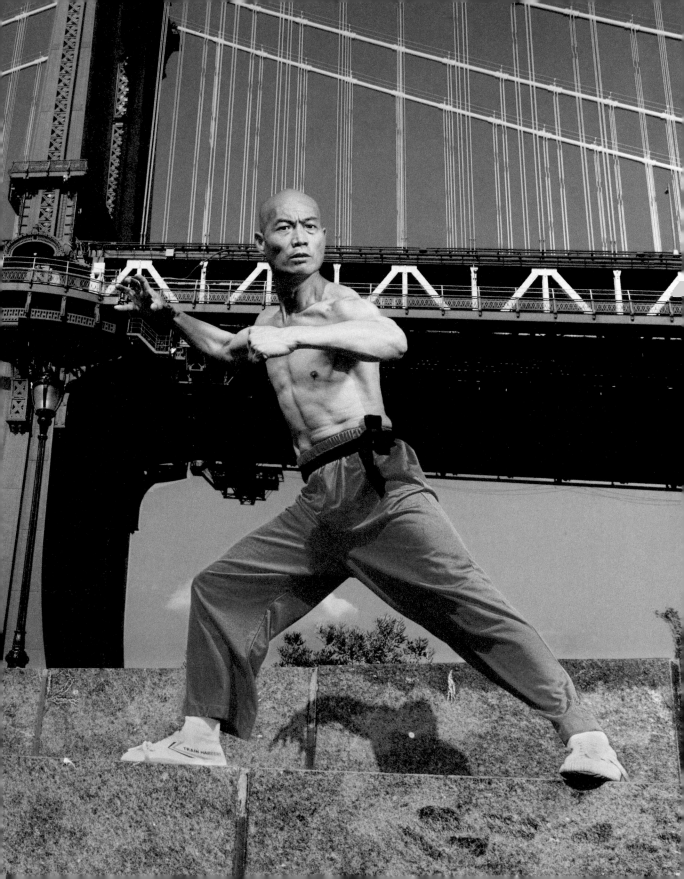

When the pressures and seductions of stardom threatened to overwhelm the shy and thoughtful rap star, he turned to training with Sifu three times a week to keep himself centered. In 1999, when Sifu made a historic return to Shaolin Temple, RZA was among the disciples who traveled there with him. Sifu was received home as a national hero. Monks from the temple, students from the area's secular kung fu schools, and many local people greeted his group at the airport with banners, drums, and cymbals. Television crews and print reporters documented the celebrations. Sifu was able to meet again with his own sifu, Yong Qian, a Grand Master of Shaolin Temple, in a reunion that deeply touched both their hearts.

But Sifu told all of his students that this historic event was not a homecoming for him alone. "Shaolin Temple is your home, too," Sifu told them. "Welcome home." To celebrate, they arranged another historic event: RZA gave the first rap performance ever at Shaolin Temple. This extraordinary meeting of cultures, of old and new traditions, beautifully encapsulated Sifu's mission to bridge the world with the principles of kung fu, or Chan Buddhism.

When the multitalented RZA decided to make his own kung-fu film, *The Z Chronicles*, he asked Sifu to star in it. On the evening when ODB, RZA's cousin, tragically died in 2004, Sifu was among the few friends RZA saw for emotional support.

Sifu sees the entertainment and media worlds as ways to help spread Shaolin Temple teaching around the world. Wesley Snipes, Rosie Perez, John Leguizamo, Bokeem Woodbine, Björk, and a number of other stars have studied under him. The guests joining Sifu's students to celebrate his 41st birthday at the temple in 2005 included Snipes, RZA, GZA, Masta Killa, filmmaker Jim Jarmusch, comedian Dave Chappelle, and pop singer Pink.

"Sifu Shi Yan Ming is a true master and a beautifully enlightened human being," Jim Jarmusch says. "Sometimes I feel enlightened just standing next to him. His physical grace and discipline are as inspiring as his finely tuned, nonjudgmental mind, and I'm deeply honored to know him."

"Sifu has crazy skills and mad science," John Leguizamo declares. "He's a philosopher-warrior straight out of the kung fu legends. I've met some world-class fighters and trainers. The great ones, like Sifu, teach that it's not just about the few minutes you might actually be in a fight someday. They show you how getting your body and your mind right can affect your whole life."

Sifu is highly respected in the action film industry, of course, where everyone from Jackie Chan to John Woo acknowledges him as a master. He has appeared in television commercials and magazine fashion spreads. He consulted on and had a brief role in Jarmusch's film *Ghost Dog: The Way of the Samurai* (featuring a superb trip-hop score by RZA). His role is a perfect illustration of how the warrior uses his kung fu skills for self-defense, not to beat people up. Sifu plays a man carrying two heavy bags of groceries who is attacked by a would-be robber. He calmly puts his

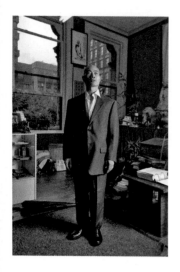

bags down and delivers two swift, precise kicks to the attacker's chest. It's done with no show of anger, and with just enough force to defend himself and scare the assailant away, not to damage him. Having defended himself, Sifu calmly picks up his bags and proceeds with his day.

He has been featured many times on national and international TV, including the National Geographic and Discovery channels, ABC, MTV, the BBC, CNBC, and TLC. He's appeared in countless newspapers and magazines around the world—among them *Time, Vibe, Entertainment Weekly,* the *New York Times, Details,* the *New Yorker,* the *Village Voice*—and of course has been on the covers of all the major kung fu and martial arts publications. He also travels to give lectures and demonstrations, finding disciples everywhere from Harvard University to elementary schools to the U.S. Naval Academy in Annapolis.

Sifu dreams of continuing the Shaolin tradition in another way. On a bright blue summer day, a National Geographic television crew accompanies him to the top of a mountain to document this vision as part of an hour-long special they are filming about him. Bear Mountain, in the Palisades Interstate Park, near West Point, is just 45 miles up the Hudson River from Manhattan. From the mountaintop you can see the city's towers glittering on the horizon like the city of Oz, yet you are surrounded by pristine nature, a panorama of rolling green hills and sparkling water, with hawks circling in the brisk, clear air overhead.

Sifu stands in his brilliant orange and yellow monk's robes on an outcropping of bald rock at the mountain's peak, with a small, wind-twisted evergreen behind him. The National Geographic crew shoots him against the blue sky and green hills as he executes a number of the stretches and strikes contained in this book. His face a stern warrior's mask, his body etching shapes as fine and precise as Chinese calligraphy, he is the very ideal of the Shaolin Temple warrior monk.

Then he sits cross-legged on a rock and describes his vision. Here in this landscape, which reminds him so much of the Song Mountains back in Henan Province, he plans to build another temple—a new Shaolin Temple—that is accessible to the metropolis of New York City yet takes advantage of the tranquil natural beauty. Here, students and disciples from around the world will be able to train in kung fu and pursue their studies of Chan Buddhism, regardless of their income or background.

Although he has lived long enough in the United States to know how hard it could be to raise the needed funds for such an undertaking, Sifu speaks with the same straightforward confidence and steadfast optimism with which he approaches all of life.

"We *will* build it," he simply says, and it's impossible to imagine that he won't.

To Sifu Shi Yan Ming, this book is yet another way to introduce people to the life transformation they may achieve through kung fu training. As with everything else he does in life, this book is a vehicle for him to help others make their bodies, minds, and lives more beautiful.

Amituofo!

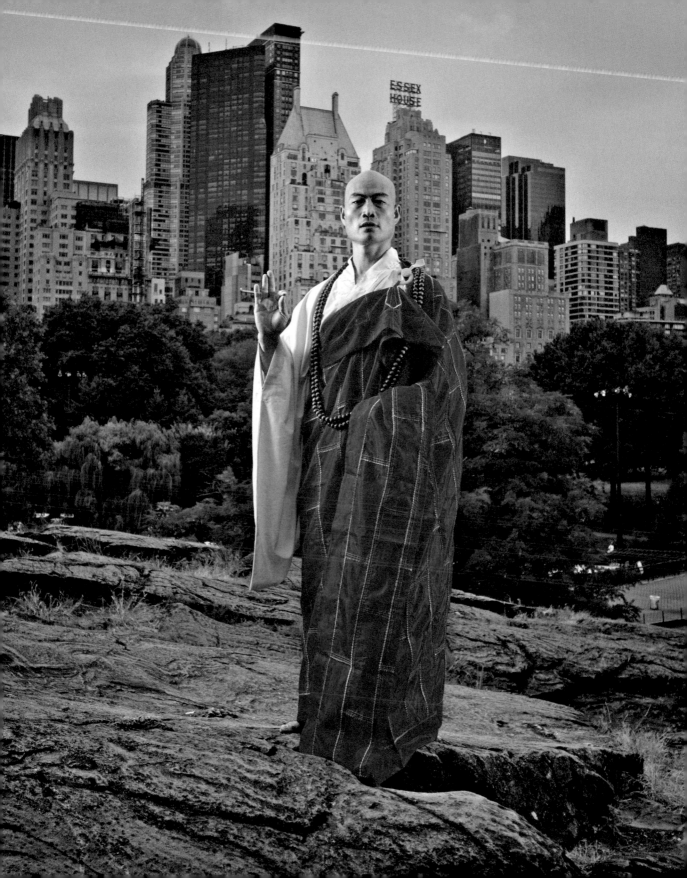

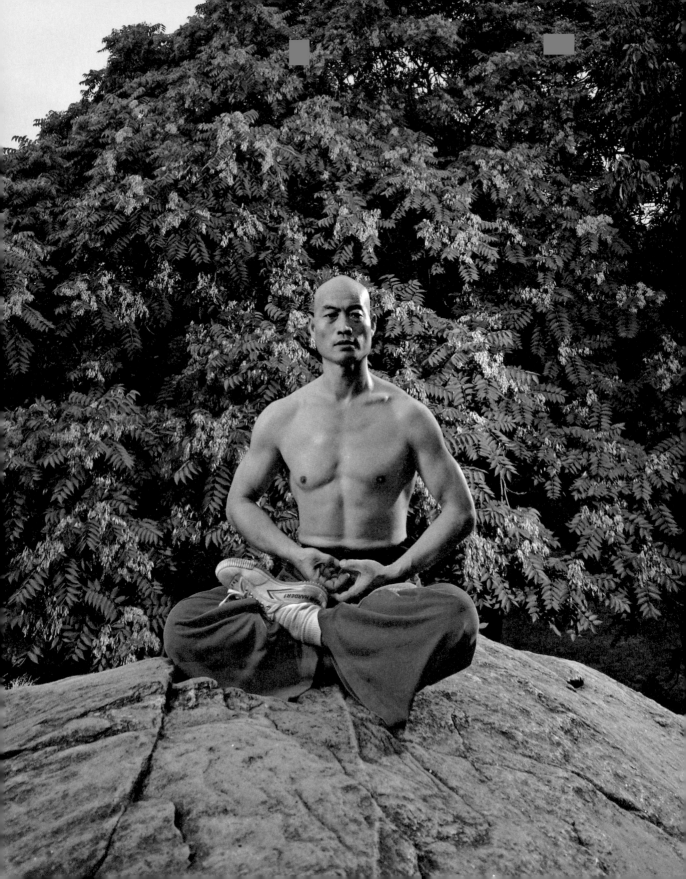

2. The Warrior's Workout

READ THIS BEFORE YOU BEGIN

Commit Yourself!

No matter how much time and effort you put into this warrior's workout, you will see benefits. But to see the best results—to really begin transforming your body and your life—you must *commit yourself* to this program. Make a promise to yourself that you will train hard and seriously, and complete the entire program. If you're just dabbling because you think it would be fun to learn a few flashy kung fu moves, you'll never get far enough into the program to learn those moves. You must follow the steps as Sifu has designed them for you. He has organized the sessions the way they are for a purpose. This will become evident to you when the stances and kicks you learn turn out to be based on fundamentals you have been practicing since the first session.

If you commit yourself and train seriously, you *will* see wonderful results. You will find that the more you train, the more you'll *want* to train. The more you put into your training, the quicker you'll master the techniques, and the more you'll change your body and your life for the better.

Keep yourself motivated by thinking seriously about the many positive messages Sifu offers. Sifu teaches: "Everyone is handsome. Everyone is beautiful." Sadly, not everyone is aware of that. This is one of the reasons we so often fail when we try to "improve" ourselves through a new exercise program or a new diet. We begin, in effect, by insulting ourselves: "I'm fat. I'm out of shape. I need to go on a diet. I need to get to the gym more often." If you start out with such a negative opinion of yourself, it's no wonder you ultimately fail. What kind of motivation is that?

As you pursue the Shaolin Workout, try to remember that you're not "improving" yourself. You don't need to be improved! God made you! You're just polishing yourself, to let your true beauty shine.

You should set aside time every day when you can focus on the training. You can complete early sessions in as little as 10 or 15 minutes. But the length of your sessions will gradually increase as you keep adding new parts to your daily workout. Eventually, you'll probably need to allot yourself ¹/₂ hour per session. Don't tell yourself you don't

31

have the time. Make the time. When you're hungry, you make time to eat, don't you? You make time when you have to go to the bathroom. This training can be no less important to your life. "If you start making excuses," Sifu says, "you'll never finish."

This training will not take time away from your kids and loved ones. In fact, you will have more energy and vitality to share with them. You will be *more* present, not less. Your training will soon become integrated and essential to your entire life.

Transform Yourself!

Sifu teaches that Chan Quan is a comprehensive physical, mental, and spiritual discipline, a way to transform your body and your whole attitude so that you can express your inner as well as your outer beauty. Along with guiding you through the fundamentals of kung fu to transform your body, the Shaolin Workout includes daily meditations that introduce you to some key concepts of Chan Buddhism. It does not tell you "everything you need to know about Chan Buddhism," and it won't turn you into a Buddhist overnight. You will gain an understanding, however, of how you can apply Sifu's philosophy of harmony and balance to improve your daily life, whatever religion or philosophy you follow.

All Buddhists believe that the world is filled with both suffering and desire, which obscure our true nature. Through meditation, they seek to clear the mind of these distractions. To Chan Buddhists, the purpose of meditation is to be fully present in the here and now, to be fully aware and mindful of *this* moment, open to the beauty of pure existence. This is not an easy state to achieve, especially in our busy modern world. Our minds are always working, processing a blizzard of input, rehashing the past, and rehearsing possible futures. In the West, when we hear the word "meditation," we tend to think only of what Sifu calls no-action meditation—sitting in stillness and quiet contemplation. This is one form of meditation. But the action meditation of Chan Quan, properly practiced, has the same effect of relaxing, clearing, and focusing the mind. The physical and mental aspects of this system are as inseparable as the head and the body. Sifu explains this integration by saying, "The philosophy is the action, and the action is the philosophy."

A central principle of Chan Buddhism is that all living creatures have Buddha inside them; all living creatures are capable of achieving enlightenment. It may take many lifetimes before one realizes one's true Buddha nature. That's one reason that every life is precious, every day is an important day, and every moment is an opportunity to understand yourself and express your true inner beauty. You should never waste a day, an hour, a minute! The action meditation of kung fu helps you develop the mental clarity, a sense of balance and harmony, so that you can live fully in the present, mindful of the beauty that is *this* moment, *this* activity, here and now.

You need not become a Buddhist to benefit enormously from the physical, mental, and spiritual transformation that you can begin to achieve through this discipline. Another fundamental tenet of Chan Buddhism is that there is no one way to enlightenment, no single religion that is correct and all others wrong. Sifu's Chan Buddhism students at the U.S.A. Shaolin Temple come from many faiths and belief systems, and he encourages them to continue going to their churches, temples, or synagogues to practice. Sifu believes that all the great spiritual leaders in history have taught the same basic truths of peace, love, and respect. Prayer is good. We all pray for the same things, whatever house of worship we're in.

There are a million doors you can go through in life. There are as many paths as there are living beings. You must choose and create your own path. Sifu sees Buddhism as a philosophy and Shaolin as a way of life. The goal is to develop "a relaxed mind in a relaxed body," enabling you to approach your entire life with more confidence, mental clarity, and an enhanced sense of respect for yourself and for others, so that the life you create expresses your true, beautiful nature.

"Stretch your body," Sifu instructs, "and you stretch your mind."

How to Train

Kung fu masters come in all sizes and body types. So do Sifu's students. No one is too young or too old, too weak or heavy, too short or too tall, to train the way of the warrior. You may think you're naturally graceful and flexible, or you may not feel that you are. It doesn't matter. Train diligently, take your time absorbing the lessons, and then apply yourself to perfecting your execution of them, and you will see wonderful results.

Some people may fear that they can't train strenuously, because they have chronic joint pain or because they've sustained a recent injury or because a doctor has advised them not to strain themselves. Of course, you should train responsibly. The purpose is to polish your body and your mind—to sharpen the blades of your body and mind—not to injure yourself. If you feel you need to take it slow at first, that's okay. Chan Quan is based on the innate harmonies and powers of your body. It also acknowledges that each and every one of our bodies is unique in its size, shape, and flexibility. While Sifu encourages you to fully extend your body in every stretch and move in the Shaolin Workout (and in your whole life), he does not ask you to overextend to the point of discomfort. When you execute a stretch or a strike, extend yourself as fully as you comfortably can today. When you repeat the same movement tomorrow, you will find that you can extend it a little farther. And a little farther the next day. As you continue to train, you will naturally feel your flexibility increasing, your joints growing suppler, and the limit to which you can comfortably extend constantly expanding.

For some stretches in the Shaolin Workout, Sifu advocates bouncing the body. Western fitness instructors often teach that bouncing (also known as "ballistic stretching") may lead to injury or muscle soreness. They can make their students afraid to move and to use their bodies. But athletes around the world use bouncing to stretch farther than they could by using static stretches, and they find it especially effective for developing muscle and tendon flexibility and speed, which are key to kung fu. Don't be afraid of your own muscles and tendons!

At the same time, no one is too fit to benefit from training this way. You may go to the gym five times a week. You may be a dedicated cyclist or Pilates enthusiast or rock climber. No matter what kind of physical training you do now, you will find that the Shaolin Workout enhances your strength, stamina, balance, and grace while transforming your mental outlook.

Though it is unique and special, the kung fu training offered in this workout requires no special clothing. Anything light and loose fitting that allows a free range of movement will do. You can train in shorts and a T-shirt, a gym outfit, or your pajamas. Many of the stretches can be executed in your street or office clothes. Just stand up from your desk and stretch the "job-related stress" out of your stiff muscles. You can execute the kicks and stances in your running shoes, socks, or bare feet. The best footwear is a pair of flexible, lightweight martial arts sneakers. Many kung fu students find these so comfortable they buy extra pairs just to walk around in.

This workout requires no equipment—your body and mind are the only tools you need. And everything in the workout can be done in a very small space. In China they say you can practice kung fu in the space a tiger lies down in. If you have a large space, a backyard or a gym where you can train, that's great. But you can train anywhere—in your bedroom, your office, a hotel room. You can get up on your desk and show off your moves to all your co-workers!

If you want to practice your stretches and movements in front of a mirror, you can. But the point is to train your body and clear your mind, so if watching yourself in the mirror is a distraction, stop doing it. Your body will know when it's doing things correctly. You'll feel it. Don't think—just do it!

The lessons are designed so that you can practice and train on your own. But if you can get someone to train with you—a spouse, child, or friend—that's fantastic. You can then observe and help each other, and you'll be enriching their lives along with your own.

Kung Fu Training and Weight Training

You do not need previous experience with any style of martial arts to successfully complete the Shaolin Workout. The majority of students who come to the U.S.A. Shaolin Temple come with no prior knowledge. In fact, because this is the pure essence of Shaolin Temple kung fu, some students who have taken other martial arts classes find that they must unlearn some incorrect practices they've been taught elsewhere.

Also, you don't need to be a "gym bunny" to become adept at kung fu. Kung fu is a very different system of exercise and strength building from Western-style bodybuilding, weight lifting, and even the typical aerobics programs we learn at the gym. The goal of Western bodybuilding, especially for men, is to build up muscle mass and sculpt it into handsome shapes. It looks great—but it doesn't move very well. In fact, bodybuilders and people who lift a lot of weights at the gym often experience problems with their joints and their backs. They can become stiff and rigidly inflexible.

Kung fu athletes tend to be trim, light, elastic, and fast. Women and men are equally competent at it. In this sense you might see some superficial resemblance to gymnasts, but because of their high-impact routines, gymnasts often experience joint and back problems that would not result from the Shaolin Workout.

Kung fu practitioners prove the simple truth that you don't need all that sculpted muscle mass to be strong. Sifu explains that there is a difference between *strength* and *power*. A very strong man may be able to lift a 500-pound boulder. That's strength. Yet what can he *do* with that rock once he's hefted it? Just hope not to drop it on his toes. But any kid can pick up a pebble and throw it a great distance. The lightness of the pebble and the speed with which the kid throws it equal power. How far can the strongest man throw that 500-pound boulder?

Here is another difference: What's the first thing that strong man does when he approaches that boulder? He starts to *think* about it. He wonders if he can lift it. He worries if he'll strain his back. He hopes he doesn't drop it on his toes. But you pick up a pebble and toss it with no thought, no pause, no worries. You don't have to think about it; you just do it. It's the most natural thing in the world.

As you train the warrior's way, you'll find that's how kung fu is. The kung fu warrior gets her power from lightness, speed, and clarity of mind. The kung fu warrior doesn't stand around thinking about how to move. She just does it, as quickly and naturally as a tiger.

There are two kinds of muscle: fast muscle and slow muscle, also known as long muscle and short muscle. The goal of Western gym training is to develop slow, short muscle. You do biceps curls slowly, tensing and bunching up that muscle. You use heavy weights, because you want to literally hurt that muscle. It remains tensed and bunched up, which is considered an attractive look. That's a muscle that cannot be used for speed and cannot be easily extended. You have trained it to move slow and tighten up. Not to mention the strain you're putting on your wrist, elbow, and shoulder.

Kung fu concentrates on fast, long muscles. It builds strength and power through speed and agility. Sifu says that whereas the goal of weight lifting is to make you thicker and bigger, kung fu extends your body and your mind, stretching them both to make them relaxed and flexible. The goal, Sifu instructs, is to stretch your body to make it 3 inches longer, not make it a foot thicker.

Look at the swiftest animals in nature—the cheetah, the leopard, the gazelle. None of them looks like a bodybuilder, with muscles bulging all over! Each of them is one long, lean, supple muscle machine, from the tip of the nose to the tip of the tail. When you watch one of them run, it looks like a single long muscle all stretched out and flexing to give the animal its incredible speed and agility. They don't go to a gym—all of nature is their gym. Finding food or eluding predators is their workout routine. Sifu never lifts weights of any kind, and of course is absolutely against the use of steroids or any drugs, and yet he is fantastically fit and amazingly powerful.

Western gym training emphasizes isolation: You work on building up one muscle or muscle group, separate from the rest of your body. If you go to the gym frequently, you probably work on your arms and shoulders one visit, your legs the next, and so on.

Chan Quan trains your entire body, from the top of your head to the tips of your toes. It emphasizes the innate harmonies of the body. It trains you to be like the tiger or the gazelle. As you progress through the Shaolin Workout, you will understand the wisdom of this approach. You will begin to feel your entire body working in beautiful coordination, not just when you're working out but all through your day—when you walk down the street, when you sit at your desk, when you bend to lift a sack of groceries. The more you train, the more you will feel all your muscles working together in this harmonious way, giving you strength and agility you may never have experienced before.

Kung fu or Chan Buddhism doesn't just extend your body; it extends your mind and spirit as well. As you train the Shaolin Workout way, committing yourself as seriously to the daily meditations as to the physical training, you will begin to develop a mental attitude that's as relaxed and poised as your transformed body. The warrior's beautiful calm and confidence will radiate throughout your entire life. That's another significant difference between Western weight lifting and Shaolin kung fu. Outside of working out at the gym or posing at the beach, the weight lifter's big muscles aren't really of much use in life. The need or even the opportunity to lift a 500-pound rock just doesn't come up very often. But the physical and mental discipline you develop through this workout can literally transform you, helping you to fully extend your life and express your beautiful being every moment of every day.

Because of all those differences, if you're accustomed to working out at a gym, you may well find yourself preferring the Shaolin Workout to your other routines. In fact, while Sifu encourages students to continue specific practices, like situps and pushups, the vast majority of people who train regularly with him give up lifting weights, Pilates, and all other exercise programs. They find that kung fu gives them a fantastic workout that's more rigorous than any aerobics class, while strengthening and making the whole body more flexible, more toned, and fitter. Kung fu constantly stimulates you with new things to learn and new ways to challenge yourself. Once you've experienced what it's like to live the warrior's way, fully extending and expressing yourself physically, mentally, and spiritually, you'll never want to limit yourself.

How the Sessions Are Organized

This workout is organized as four 1-week parts containing 7 sessions each. In the first week, you learn basic stretches and warmup exercises, along with daily philosophical meditations that will stretch your mind the same way you're stretching your body. These early sessions increase your flexibility and balance, both physically and metaphysically, which are essential to kung fu. Also, they are the building blocks that you will combine in different ways when you execute the stances, strikes, and kicks you will learn in the following weeks.

In each session, you are instructed to practice everything you've learned in previous sessions. Do not skip over this practice and jump straight to the new lesson. You're only cheating yourself. The daily stretches warm up your muscles and joints so that you can perform better and with less possibility of an accident or a pulled muscle.

Relatively speaking, the lessons increase in complexity as you progress through the parts. You will probably find the early stretches easier to learn and execute than some of the beautifully orchestrated movements you'll learn toward the end of the program. But don't worry if even some of the early stretches seem hard at first. If everyone could master all of kung fu right off the bat, the world would be full of Sifus. Don't give up if you find a stretch or stance hard—train harder! In China, there is a saying: "Don't be afraid of going slowly. Be afraid only of standing still." Apply yourself, train regularly with discipline and confidence, and you *will* see improvement. You *will* master the moves, and pretty soon you'll be beautifully executing a stretch or stance that seemed difficult when you first tried it. This is another reason daily repetition is built into the program. Your body and muscles learn through repetition.

In the daily meditations, Sifu gives you the tools to develop the mental clarity and self-confidence to stick with the training and master every move. It can't be overstressed that these mental and spiritual exercises are as essential as the physical ones, and the two are inseparably linked. When you approach every task with a warrior's relaxed and focused mind, you will find that there's nothing you can't do. Only you can limit yourself. Kung fu or Chan Buddhism offers you keys to unlock your unlimited power.

The Shaolin Workout adds something new for you to learn every day, except for the last day of each week, which is set aside for you to review and practice everything you've already learned. Ideally, you will be able to complete the training in 28 consecutive days. If, however, you find a specific stance or kick simply too complex to learn in a single session, do *not* give up on that lesson and simply jump ahead to the next. It's better to deviate from the schedule if you must and spend an extra day or two getting that movement down than to give up on it and go on to the next move.

Think of it as being like learning a new language. When you first start out, learning another language can seem very hard. All the words are unfamiliar to you. At first, you have to stop and think every time you open your mouth to speak this new language. You have to learn ways to express yourself that are different from the ones you've been using naturally and without a thought all your life. Then, as you continue to learn and practice it, a wonderful transformation naturally occurs. The new words just come to you, without your having to stop and think of them. They begin to fall into place in the right order to build sentences. Gradually, you become more fluent, until your new language flows as easily and naturally as the one you grew up speaking.

As you progress in this workout, you'll find the same thing happening. As you train, you will become more fluent, expressing yourself through beautiful movements that flow naturally and without a thought. As you keep exercising your mind as well as your body, the self-respect and self-confidence you develop will inspire you to see each new lesson as an exciting opportunity to learn and extend yourself further. The truth is, as we said before, the more you train, the more you'll want to train, the more you'll enjoy training, and the more you'll get out of it in ways that will benefit your entire life.

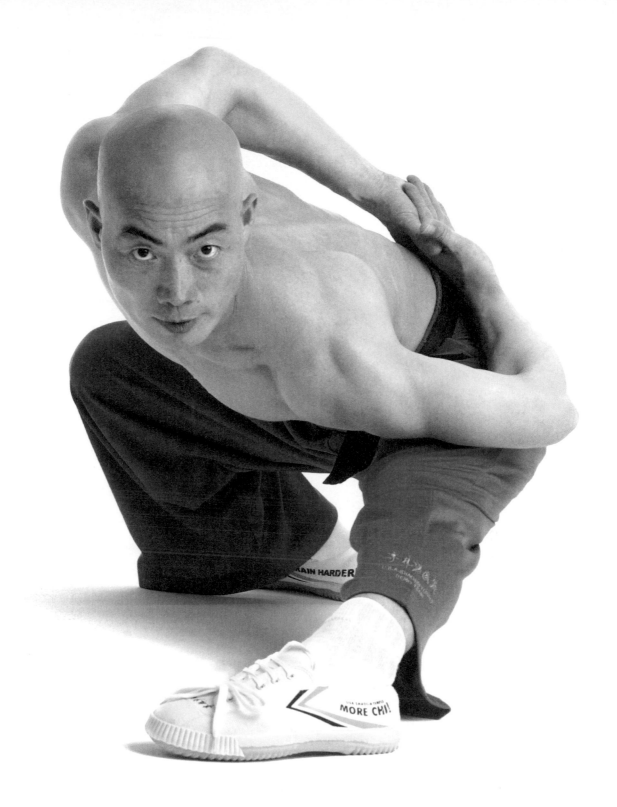

THE SHAOLIN WORKOUT

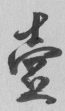

PART ONE

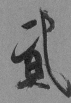

PART TWO

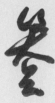

PART THREE

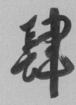

PART FOUR

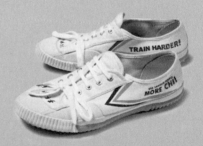

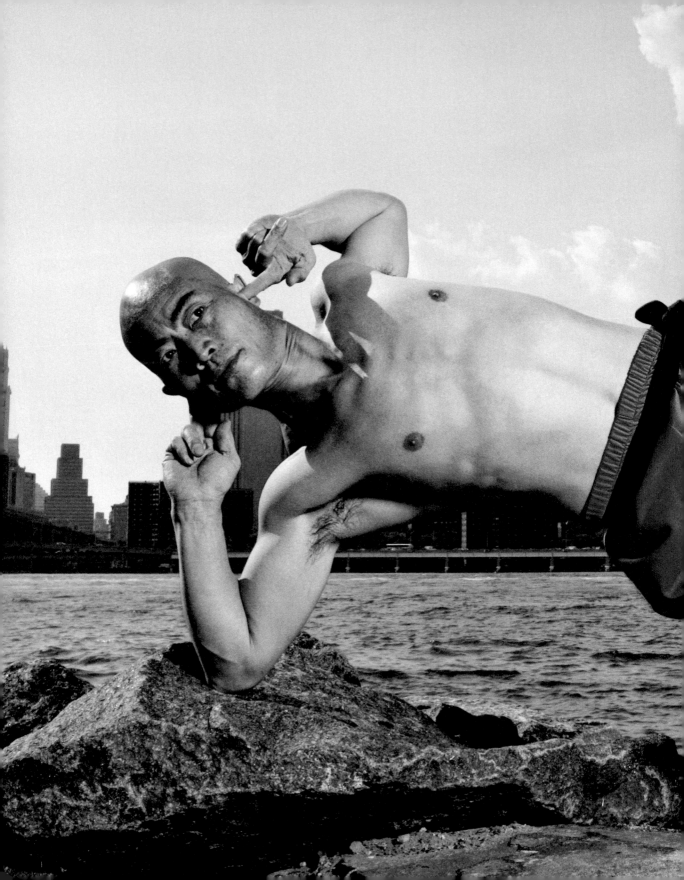

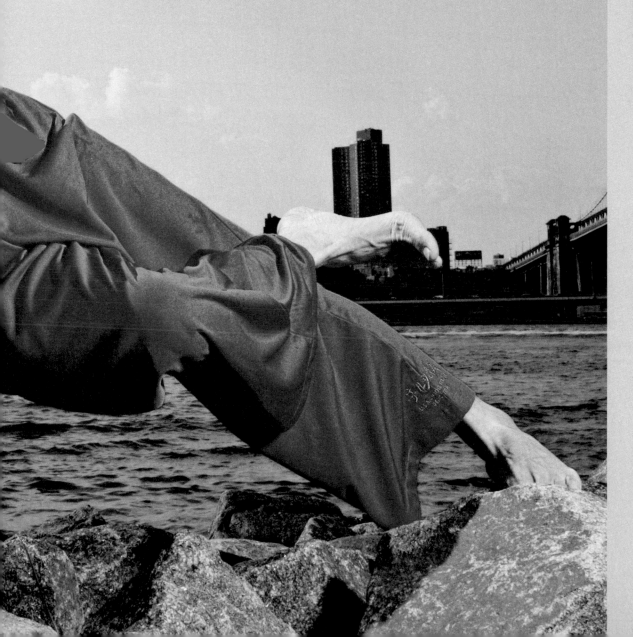

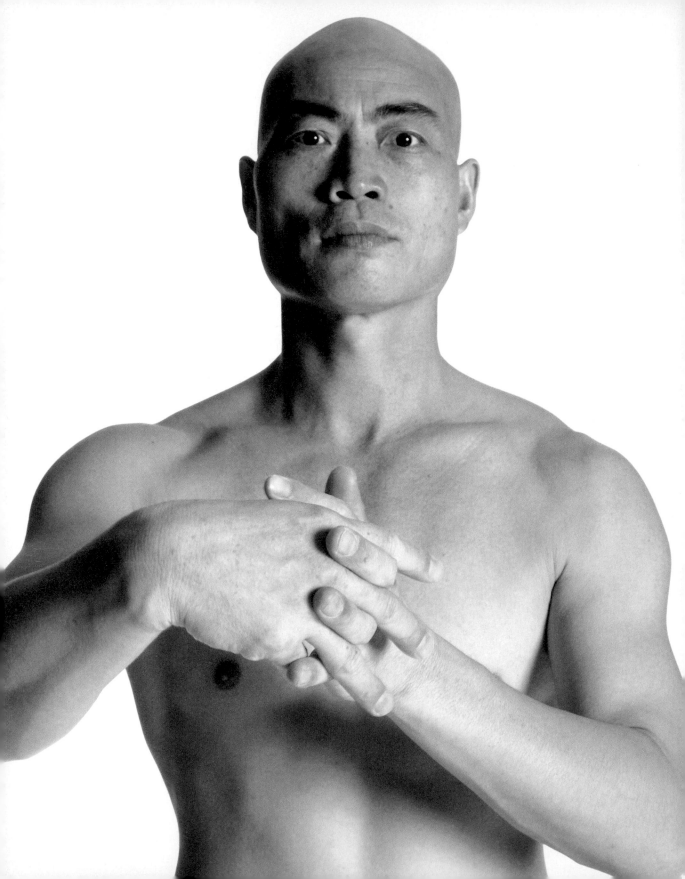

Wrists and Ankles

**Welcome to your first day of the Shaolin Workout,
the program Sifu Shi Yan Ming has specially designed for you.**

As you train way of the warrior, Sifu says, "You may feel sore, you may feel pain, you may feel sour, you may feel sweet. But you will also feel the most fabulous and enjoyable feelings you ever had."

At the U.S.A. Shaolin Temple, we begin and end every session with chanting the name of one of the Buddhas, Amituofo, pronounced *ah-mee-toh-foh*. Try it at home, or wherever you'll be doing this training. Call it out like a joyous cheer, "AH-MEE-TOH-FOH!" Repeat it three times.

The first time is to pay respect to Buddha.

The second time is for the Dharma, the way of life.

The third time is to pay respect to Sifu, the Master. At home, master yourself. Encourage yourself. More chi! Train harder!

WRIST ROTATION

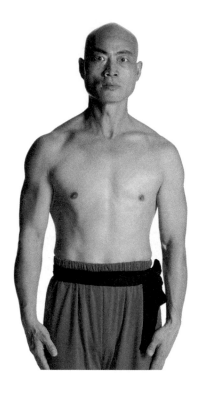 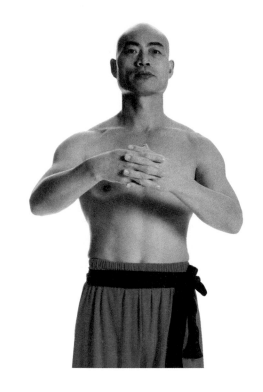

Stand straight and relaxed, with your feet comfortably apart, slightly wider than your shoulders. And right here, at the start of your very first lesson, learn the most important principle of all martial arts training: extension. Throughout your training, and throughout your life, fully extend your body. Stand tall. Stretch your spine and reach for the sky with the top of your head. Hold your chin high, and square your shoulders. Open your chest to the world, and open your heart to the world's limitless beauty.

Extension is absolutely key to your transformation. When your body and your mind are fully extended and relaxed, you will get the most out of your training. And the same is true of your life. If you're not relaxed in mind and body, you can't fully enjoy your beautiful life. Fully extend your body and extend your mind, and you extend your whole life.

Hold your hands out in front of your chest, elbows bent, palms toward you, thumbs toward the sky. Lace your fingers. Now rotate your wrists in a winding, curling motion, rolling your wrists outward. Really stretch your wrists outward with each turn, extending fully. Make circles in the air with your wrists. Think of the Buddhist Wheel of Life.

Don't worry if it feels a little awkward at first. Relax. Loosen up. It feels good, doesn't it?

Do it 10 times. Count it out. In fact, since you are training the Shaolin Workout way, you might as well learn a little

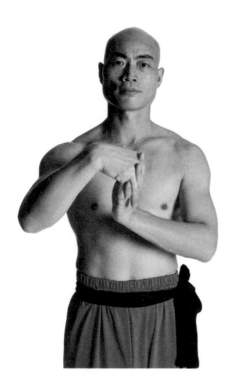

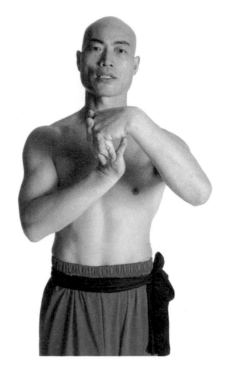

Chinese as well. Here's how to count to 10 in Mandarin Chinese as it is spoken in Henan Province, home of the Shaolin Temple:

Yi (pronounced *yee*)
Er (ehr)
San
Si (suh)
Wu
Liu (lyoo)
Qi (chee)
Ba
Jiu (jyoo)
Shi (sher)

Now reverse the direction of the rotation. Roll your wrists toward you. Repeat 10 times. Count it out.

Excellent! You've completed your first Shaolin Workout exercise!

ANKLE ROTATION

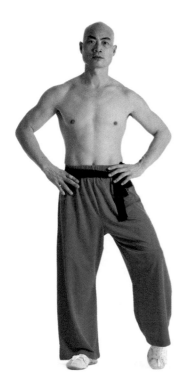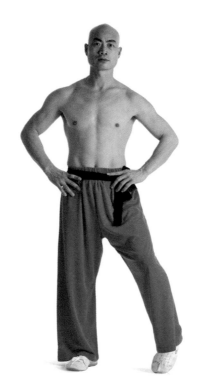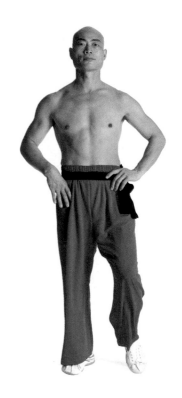

Stand straight and relaxed, fully extended. Lift your left foot onto its toes. Bend your knee enough so that you're stretching and extending your whole foot and ankle and balancing your foot on the tips of your toes. You'll feel the stretch in your calf as well. When you stretch your body, you stretch your mind, too.

Rotate your ankle in a clockwise direction. Make sure to keep your foot and ankle fully extended. Do it 10 times. Count it out: *yi, er, san, si, wu, liu, qi, ba, jiu, shi.*

Reverse the direction, rotating your ankle in a counter-clockwise direction. Do it 10 times.

Now do the right foot. Rotate clockwise 10 times and then counterclockwise.

COMBINED WRIST AND ANKLE ROTATION

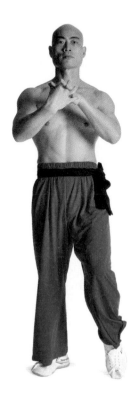

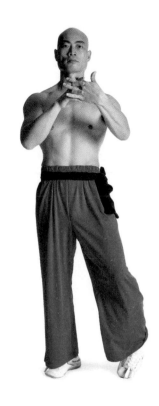

Now combine those first two exercises, rotating your wrists and one ankle at the same time. Don't worry if it seems a bit complicated at first, like rubbing your stomach and patting your head at the same time. You'll get it. Relax your body and mind. Don't think about it—just do it!

Rotate your wrists forward while rotating the left foot clockwise. Count to 10.

Reverse the direction. Roll your wrists toward you while rotating your left ankle counterclockwise. Do it 10 times.

Now for the right ankle. Roll the wrists forward while rotating the right foot clockwise. Then reverse: Roll your wrists toward you while rotating your right ankle counterclockwise.

Magnificent!

Meditation

More chi! Train harder!

Sifu often encourages his students with the cheer "More chi! Train harder!"

What does this mean?

Chi (also spelled qi) is often translated as "life force." It is similar to what we in the West mean by "energy," but it's much more than that. Chi is the vital force that flows through all things—humans, animals, plants, rocks, microbes, mountains. Chi connects us to all other things in the universe. It is the source of all spiritual, mental, and physical energy and health. It is dynamic, circulating in us like our blood. It has been compared to electricity flowing through circuits, and to the force flowing around magnetic poles.

When our minds, hearts, and bodies are in harmony and in balance, the chi flows freely, helping us to live beautiful lives. When our lives are out of balance, the chi may be blocked or depleted. Stimulating the correct flow of chi can heal us when we are sick and invigorate us when we are tired.

Chi is the force that gives kung fu masters like Sifu their incredible power. It is through stimulating and guiding the flow of chi that we train and push our bodies to actions we might never have known we could do before. This is why we constantly cheer one another on with the cry "More chi! Train harder!" The more chi you put into your exercises and movements, the harder you are able to train. The harder you train, the more you master your body and its movements, and the more chi you'll have.

Some beginners fear that they'll never be able to master certain stretches or movements. It's not unusual to experience some muscle pain when first performing certain exercises and stretches. A "pulled muscle" is a muscle that's not used to being stretched and worked. In the modern world, we use our legs for so little. We sit all day in our cars, at our desks, on the sofa, watching TV. Now you're suddenly asking your muscles to do some work. It's no wonder they're sore!

The *wrong* way to respond to that sore muscle is to tense up, physically or mentally. Tension will only block the flow of chi to that muscle.

The *right* way to respond is to relax your body and your mind, extend your body and your mind, and train harder. Athletes have that saying, "No pain, no gain." That's what "Train harder!" means as well. Don't back away from the work, don't tense up, and certainly don't give up. If you give up on your exercises, you give up on yourself. Have faith and confidence in yourself, and tomorrow the stretch you found difficult will feel easier. The next day, it will be easier still.

Today, think about how you can apply this warrior's attitude to your whole life. The more chi you put into your life, the more you'll get out of your life. When you feel like you just can't face another day of washing and folding the kids' laundry . . . when your boss drops an extra stack of paperwork on your desk an hour before quitting time . . . when you get home exhausted after fighting rush hour and plop down on the sofa, and your son asks you to help him with his math homework. Whatever chores, problems, or responsibilities you face today, don't flinch from them, don't avoid them, don't feel defeated by them. Tackle them head-on. Put more chi into it and get it done. Train harder!

Congratulations! You've completed your first training session. Now end your session with this chant:

"AMITUOFO! AMITUOFO! AMITUOFO!"

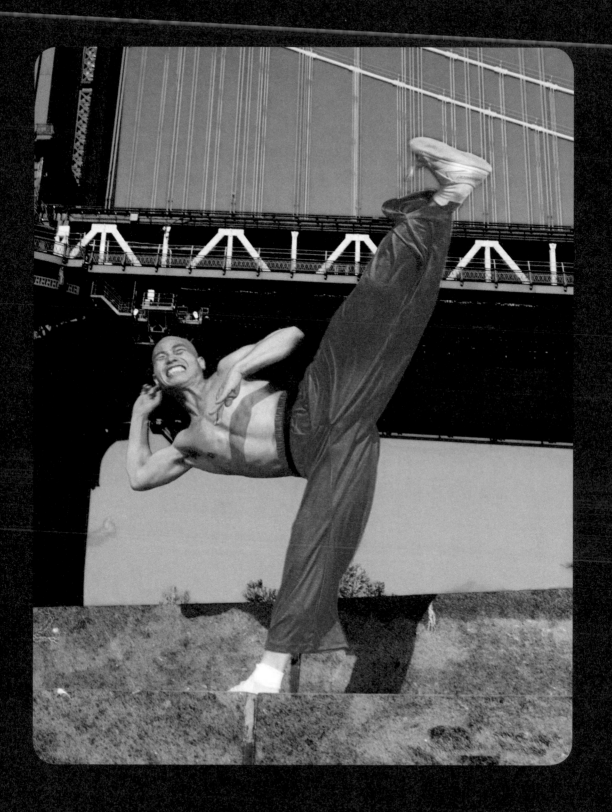

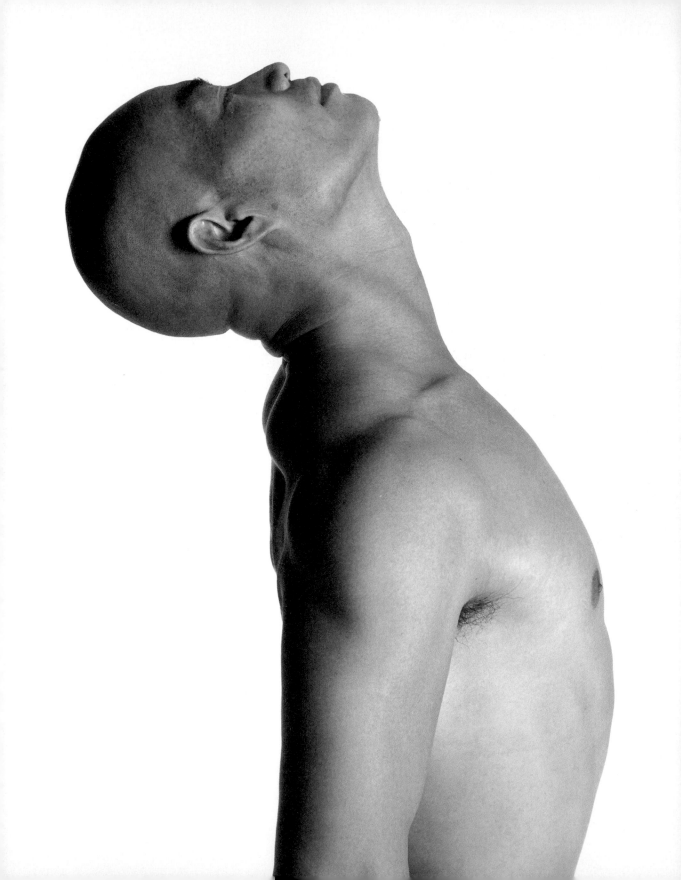

Neck and Eyes

"AMITUOFO!"
"AMITUOFO!"
"AMITUOFO!"

Remember to begin each session by building on the previous days.

In China they say, "*Wen gu er zhixin*" (溫故而知新)—practicing old things is the same as learning new ones. Today, begin by practicing what you learned yesterday. Do the wrist and ankle exercises. Wrists first, then left ankle, then right ankle, then combined. Forward 10 times; then reverse 10 times. Remember to fully extend your body and relax your mind.

Because so many of us spend so much time sitting and hunching forward—at the computer, at the wheel of the car—our bodies build up a lot of tension and tightness in our necks and shoulders. Neck stretches and rotations release that tension.

NECK STRETCH

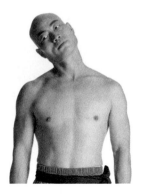 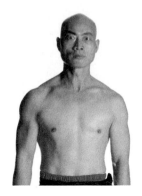 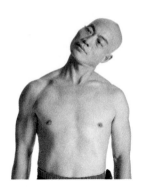

Stand straight and relaxed, fully extended, feet together, with your hands at your sides. Slowly tilt your head to one side.

Let's begin to the right. Don't turn your head—keep your face forward. As you stretch your neck by tilting your head to the right, extend your left shoulder, using the power of opposites. You'll feel the stretch down your neck and through your left shoulder and even down your left

side. Let your head's own weight carry it toward your right shoulder so your right ear is facing your shoulder, your left ear to the sky, your face forward. Hold it as fully extended as you can and count to 10. Stretch your muscles, and you stretch your mind.

Bring your head back upright, pause a second, and then tilt it to the left. Fully extend your neck and your right shoulder. Hold it for a count of 10.

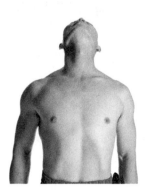 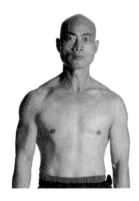 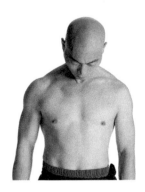

Bring your head back upright. Now let it fall slowly backward. Extend your neck until you're looking up at the sky. Don't overarch your back; just keep your body fully extended and let your neck stretch your head back as far as it can. Hold it for a count of 10. You'll feel the stretch in your whole body.

Bring your head back upright. Now tilt it forward. Let it fall slowly toward your chest and fully extend your neck so that you're looking straight down at your toes. Hold it there for a count of 10. Feel it stretching your back and shoulders.

Outstanding.

NECK ROTATION

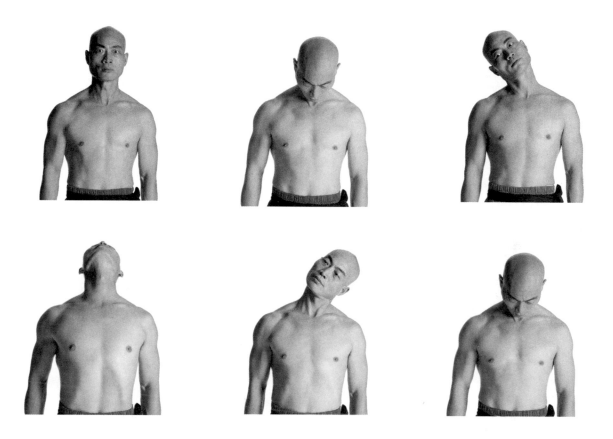

Continue to loosen up the neck. Stand straight and relaxed, your body fully extended and your mind relaxed.

Let your head fall forward, toward your chest. Don't lift your shoulders; just let your head lower itself and your neck muscles do the stretching. Extend the neck fully, until you're looking straight down at your toes.

Rotate your head, making a wide circle. In one slow, smooth, circular motion, move your head around to your right shoulder; then let it fall back until you're looking at the sky; then continue to bring it around to the left, and complete the circle by letting your chin come around toward your chest again, until you're back where the circle started, looking at your toes. Don't turn your body as your head makes its circle—remain standing straight and fully extended, chest forward. Repeat 10 times.

Excellent! Note how much better and more relaxed your neck feels.

EYE FOCUS

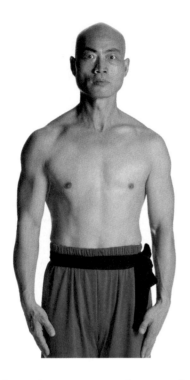 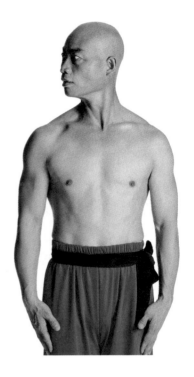

We often forget that our eyes, too, have muscles. We don't "stretch" our sight the way we do other muscles. Walking down the street, we tend to look just a few feet in front of us. We don't raise our heads and look far down the street. Our eyes passively gather information from close up. We don't reach out with our eyes to embrace the world.

We spend so much time speaking into telephones, we forget how important eye contact is in one-on-one conversation. Sifu does not like to use the telephone. He much prefers direct eye-to-eye contact. Eye to eye means mind to mind, heart to heart.

Strong eyes are of utmost importance to the warrior. Have you ever watched a lion or tiger on television, stalking and then bursting upon its prey? It leads the attack with its eyes. All the rest of its magnificent body follows its eyes as it watches sharply, calculating speed and distance, supremely focused, and then explodes across the distance between it and its goal. The eyes are critical to its power.

Sifu says the fist is like a shooting star, and the eye is like a sword. This exercise is designed to keep our eyes honed and sharp. Later in the Shaolin Workout program, you'll be glad you've been doing this training, because sharply turning your head and eyes left and right is an integral part of many moves.

Stand fully extended and relaxed, hands at sides, facing forward.

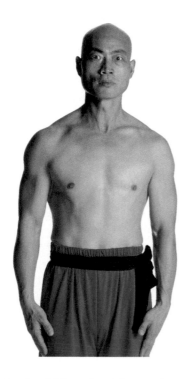

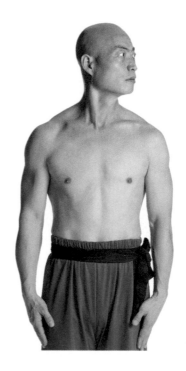

Snap your head quickly to the right, turning a full 90 degrees, so that your chin is over your shoulder, and focus your eyes as far into the distance as possible. Snap your head back straight. Now snap it to the left, look far, and snap your head straight again. Do this one quickly. Boom—left. Bam—straight. Boom—right. Bam—straight. Don't turn your body. Stand fully extended, with your feet planted firmly on the ground and your chest forward.

Even if you're standing in your bedroom and can only see the wall a few feet away, project your vision farther than that. At the U.S.A. Shaolin Temple, Sifu instructs students to see as far as Iceland and its polar bears in one direction, and as far as Miami and its dolphins in the other. Always

extend your sight as far as you can, or you won't be able to see your beautiful future! Fully extend your sight, just as you fully extend your mind, your body, and your whole life.

Do it 10 times, quick.

Awesome! Feel it in your neck muscles? Today you'll probably notice that you're carrying your head higher and lighter than before, chin up, meeting the world eye to eye. It's a nice feeling, isn't it? It's a small but important change in your posture, which you will find having a positive effect on your whole attitude, your whole way of facing the world. And people around you will notice, too.

Meditation

As I go through my day today, I will remind myself to relax. Stay loose.
Be flexible in my body and mind.

It's most important to stay loose and relaxed in mind and body. To enjoy your life, you must be relaxed. When we were children, our bodies were loose, relaxed, and flexible. We could do splits, flips, jumps, and twists without thinking about it. We were pure mind in babies' bodies.

But you're never too old—we just get too tense, too stiff. We think too much. One of the most important lessons you can learn doing the Shaolin Workout is how to get back that childlike relaxation and flexibility—to be at home in your body again. It makes no difference if you are in your twenties, fifties, or eighties. Relax. Never feel old. Tell yourself you're not getting older every year—you're getting younger!

Sifu explains that there are two kinds of meditation: action meditation and no-action meditation. In the West, we're most familiar with the no-action kind. We can all form images of Buddhist monks sitting with their legs crossed and their eyes closed, still and silent, for hours and hours, as they strive to achieve enlightenment.

The only problem is that too much no-action meditation can be as bad for your joints, your back, your neck, as sitting at a computer all day. This is what Da Mo saw happening to the monks at Shaolin. They spent so much time sitting in meditation that their bodies were as stiff as wooden dolls. He saw that Ba Tuo had not given them the proper tools to adapt Buddhism to Chinese life. Why do we meditate? To cleanse our minds and open our hearts. But if we burden our bodies with tension and pain, our minds and hearts can't be cleansed. Your mind and your heart and your body are inseparable.

Kung fu is action meditation. The goal of kung fu is to relax your body and your mind, to extend your body and your mind, to cleanse your body and your mind. To be relaxed in your body, and relaxed in your life, is how you live fully in the present, experiencing *this* moment, here and now.

In our modern world, there's another benefit to action meditation. We all have lives, jobs, families. We have wonderful things coming into our lives every day. Who among us has the time to sit and meditate for hours a day, like monks in a monastery? As you'll find out, a half-hour of action meditation can be as liberating, for your body and your mind and your heart, as several hours of no-action meditation.

Kung fu and martial arts represent a refined form of action meditation. But any exercise program can be a form of action meditation—running, swimming, playing tennis, riding a bike. In the West, we speak of that point in an exercise routine where we "get in the zone," where we "release endorphins," where we achieve "the runner's high." Those are all Western ways of approaching the same concept: action meditation. A relaxed mind in a relaxed body.

As you go through your day today, relax. Stay loose. Be flexible in your body and in your mind. Enjoy your beautiful life every minute of the day.

"AMITUOFO! AMITUOFO! AMITUOFO!"

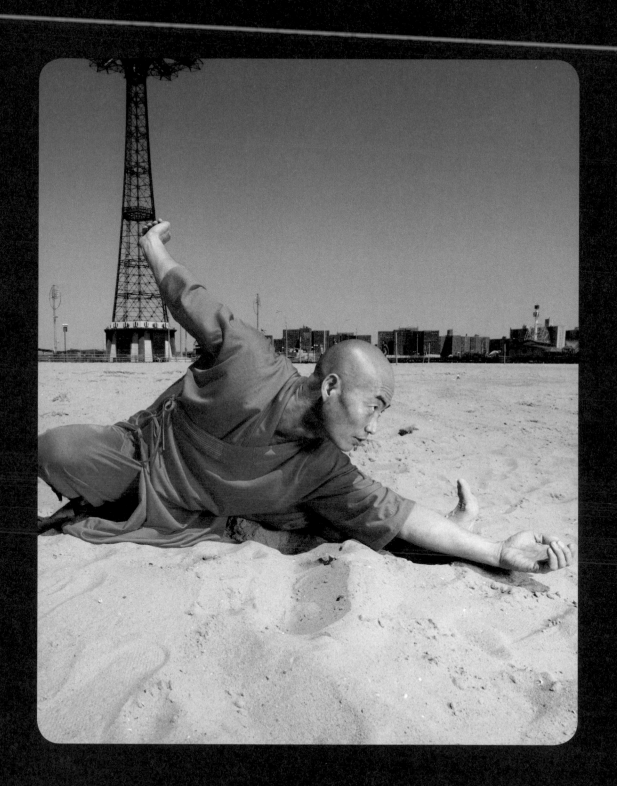

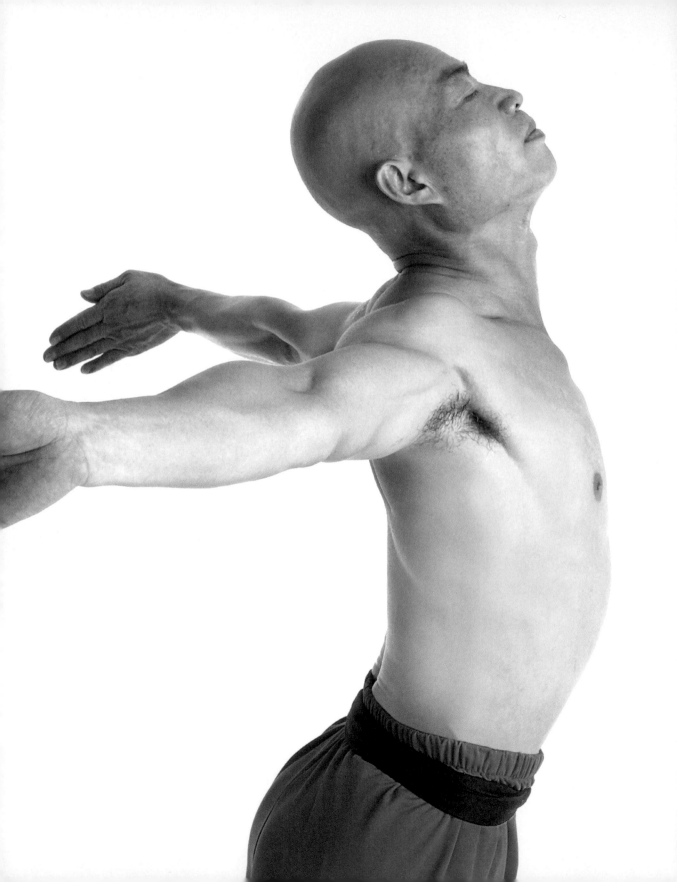

SESSION 3
Shoulders, Arms, and Chest

"AMITUOFO!"
"AMITUOFO!"
"AMITUOFO!"

Begin by going through the previous six exercises.

Today we're learning exercises that stretch and loosen the upper body. You'll be very pleased with the way they make you feel and look. Very soon you'll find yourself standing and sitting more upright, shoulders square, head up, facing the world, your body and mind fully extended.

SHOULDER ROTATION

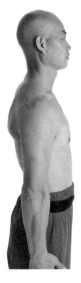 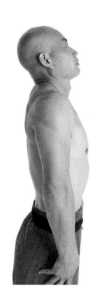 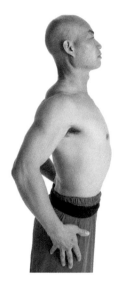 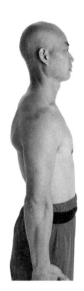

Stand relaxed and fully extended, feet comfortably apart. Hold your palms flat in front of your thighs—not gripping your thighs, just resting flat.

Slowly roll your shoulders forward, then down, then back, then up, in one circular motion. Keep the rest of your body fully extended. You'll feel your shoulder and upper-back muscles stretching and loosening with that very first rotation. Do it with energy. Extend fully. Repeat it 10 times. Count it out: *yi, er, san, si* . . .

Great. Now reverse the direction. Roll your shoulders up, back, down, and forward, making a complete circle. Repeat 10 times.

ARM STRETCH

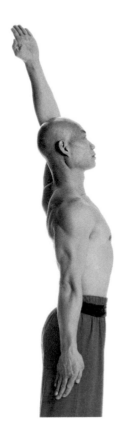
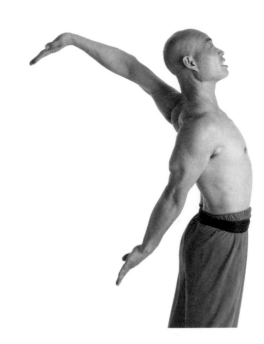

Now that you've loosened up your shoulders, do the arms.

Stand straight and relaxed, fully extended, with your feet slightly wider than your shoulders.

Lift one arm—for this example, make it the left arm—straight up, fully extended, palm forward, fingers pointing to the sky. Keep your arm close to your head. Really stretch and extend, as though you're trying to reach the sky with your fingertips. Your right arm, meanwhile, is straight down at your side, palm facing backward, fingers pointing down. Don't bend your body or your knees—stay at full extension.

Now, in a quick, sharp motion, push both your hands behind you at the same time. Don't windmill your arms—that's the next exercise. Just push and stretch your arms and shoulders behind you. Do it with chi. Use your whole, fully extended body and really give it some bounce, throwing your chest forward as you push your arms back. Do it 10 times, counting it out with chi: *Yi! Er! San! Si!* You'll feel the stretch all the way from your shoulders down through your chest and stomach to your groin and hips.

Now reverse. Lift your right arm straight up, and hold your left arm straight down, and push back in quick, sharp motions, 10 times.

ARM ROTATION

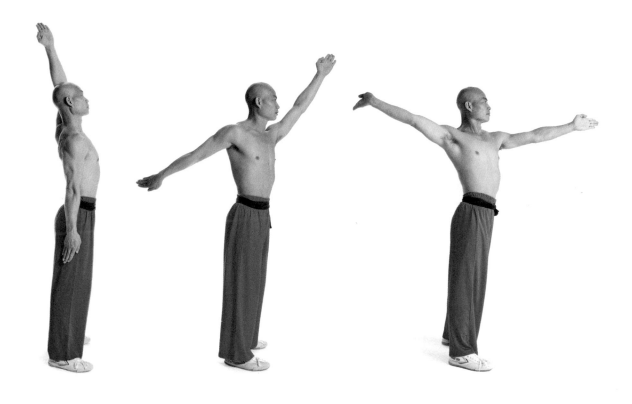

Continue working the arms and shoulders. Start in the same position as in the arm stretch: left arm straight up, palm forward, fingers reaching for the sky, right arm straight down at your side, fingers pointing down. Fully extend.

Now move your arms like the blades of a propeller, rotating the left arm forward and down at the same time you're rotating the right arm back and up. Rotate them in full, wide, alternating circles, like you're doing windmills. Keep your arms straight and close to your body as you

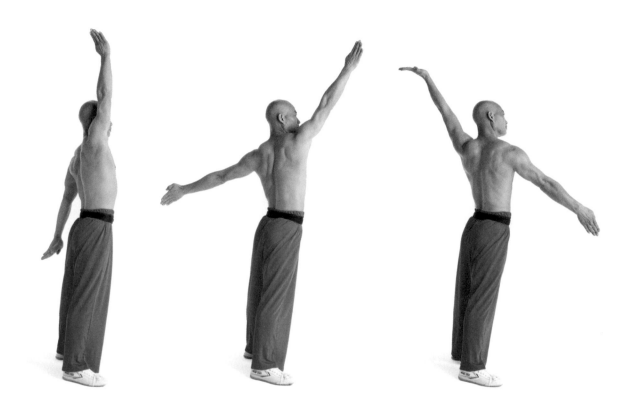

rotate them. Do it with speed and chi, counting out 10 full rotations. Ultimately, you will rotate your arms with such speed and chi that you'll feel the blood pumping all the way to your fingertips.

Now reverse the direction, rotating backward instead of forward. Repeat 10 times.

Fantastic! Your posture is better already.

OPEN CHEST

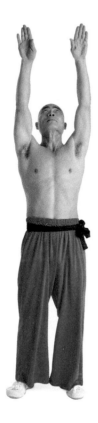 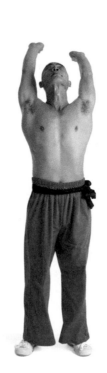 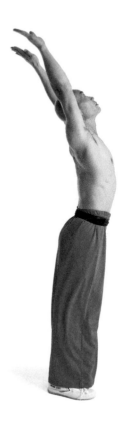

Stand straight and fully extended, with your feet slightly wider apart than your shoulders.

Stretch both arms straight up toward the sky, palms forward. Look straight ahead. Really extend—reach for the sky with your fingertips. Push your hands back simultaneously in one quick motion, really stretching and fully extending. Put your whole, fully extended body into it. Open your chest, and open your heart. Accept new things in the universe. Do it 10 times. You're toning muscles from your chest down through your groin. Soon you'll develop what kung fu masters call Iron Groin!

OPEN ARMS

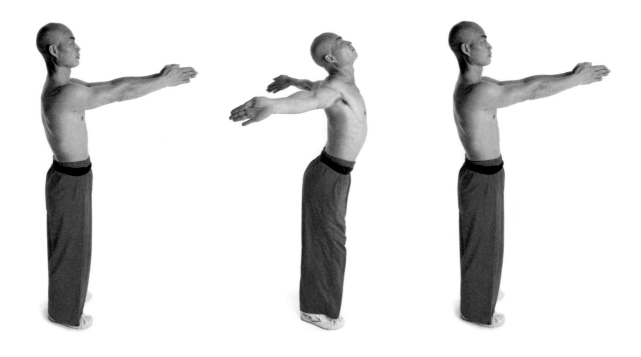

Stand fully extended, with your feet comfortably apart. Lift your arms straight out in front of you at shoulder height, fully extended, and touch your palms together. Look straight ahead.

Fling your arms open as wide as you can, as though you're throwing your arms open to embrace the universe. Your hands should be perpendicular to the ground, fingers together. Don't just open your arms—fling them open with joyful energy. Really snap them open. Pop! Throw your chest open. Turn yourself inside out!

Snap your arms back to the starting position, palms touching.

Repeat 10 times. Count it out. You'll feel your chest muscles stretching and opening with each and every count.

Spectacular! Feel how you're standing straighter and taller? Feel the confidence? Do you know how gorgeous you look right now? How handsome?

Meditation

If I want to do it, nothing is difficult. If I don't want to do it, nothing is easy.

There are rooms at Shaolin Temple where visitors can see odd indentations in the stone walls and stone grounds—hollows where the stones look like they've been worn away by years and years of repeated blows.

They have been. At times when the practice of kung fu was forbidden, monks trained at night and in secrecy in these rooms. The indentations in the walls are the spots where they practiced and practiced and practiced their fist strikes. The worn places in the stone ground are spots where they stomped their feet over and over, practicing Xin Yi Quan (heart and mind fist), and wore the stones down with years of repetition.

There's a good reason for all this practice, practice, practice, repeat, repeat, repeat. It's one thing to learn a movement with your head—to read about it, study the photos, and say, "Yes, I see. I get it." Then your body has to learn it. And your body learns through action, by doing a move over and over and over until it's completely natural and instinctive.

Like the stretches you learned today. You'll see over the next several days that as you keep practicing them, keep repeating them, your mind and your body will become one in the action. You won't have to think about them. Your muscles will just do them, because they've learned the moves.

Athletes know the truth of this. So do musicians and dancers. How do you get to Carnegie Hall? Exactly.

You can apply this to your entire life. Nothing is difficult or easy in itself. You make it difficult or easy on yourself. There's nothing you can't learn to do, if you really want it. If you want to do it, nothing is difficult. If you don't want to do it, nothing is easy. Normally, when you're thirsty, there's nothing easier than getting yourself a glass of water. Then again, when you wake up in the middle of the night thirsty, it suddenly seems difficult. You have to get up, find your slippers, trudge to the kitchen, open the fridge. . . .

Students will sometimes say to Sifu, "Sifu, I need your advice. I just can't do this move."

"You already answered yourself," Sifu replies. "You already closed your mind and limited yourself. If you say you can't do it, you won't."

In kung fu they say that the master opens the door; then the student must go through it on his or her own: *"Sifu ling jin men, xiuxing zai geren"* (師父領進門, 修行再個人). In the Shaolin Workout, Sifu gives you the knowledge; then you must train yourself. If you really want to master these skills, you will. Never tell yourself you can't do it. Just keep training and practicing. You'll be getting better every day.

"AMITUOFO! AMITUOFO! AMITUOFO!"

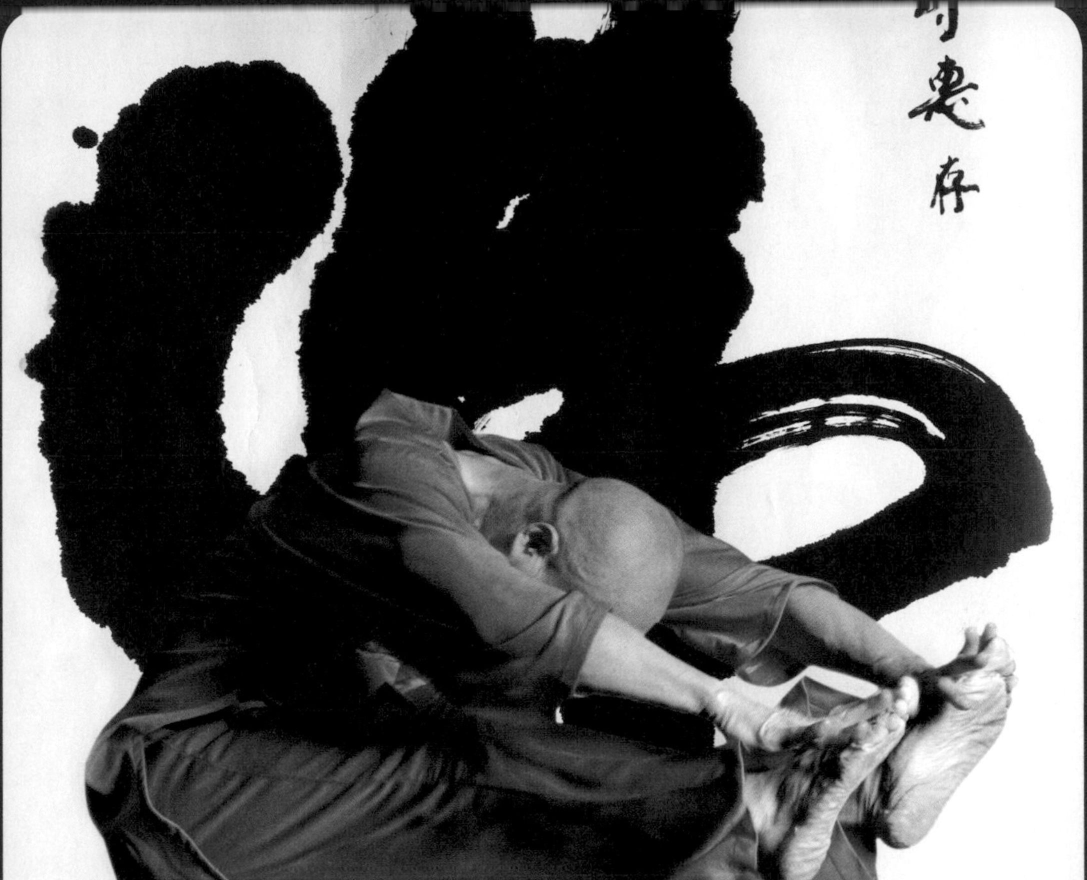
惠存
佛曆二五四三年
嵩山少林大禪

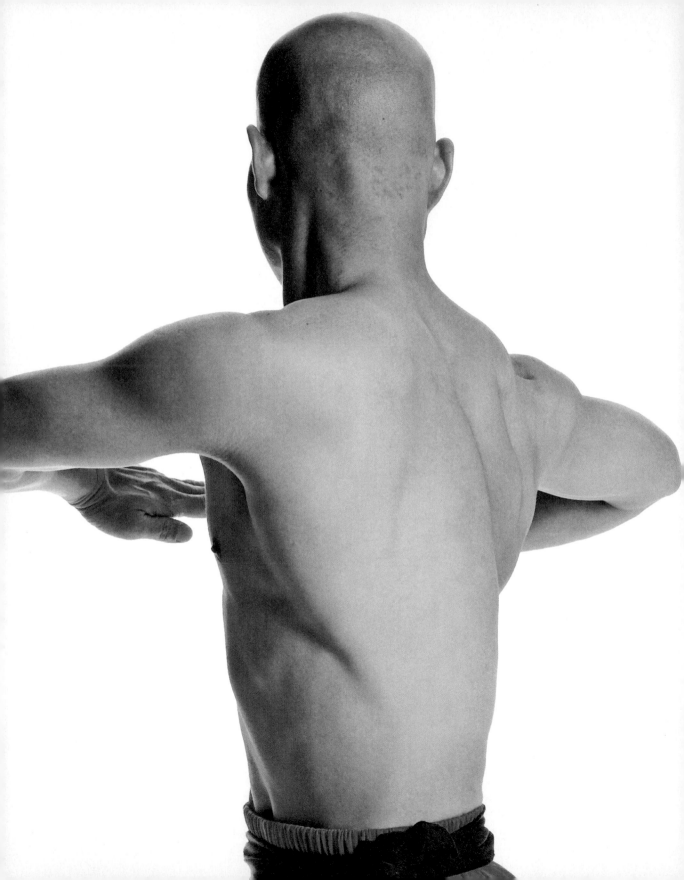

SESSION 4
Waist and Stomach

"AMITUOFO!"

"AMITUOFO!"

"AMITUOFO!"

**Begin by doing the previous 11 exercises, left and right,
forward and reverse, 10 times each.**

By now you should find you're doing most of them with increasing ease and speed. You're improving every day! Cheer yourself on. More chi! Train harder!

Today we'll stretch the waist and stomach. The waist is the center of your body. If your waist is flabby and heavy, you feel it in the rest of your body—the extra stress on your lower back, the extra weight on your knees. Sifu says that a strong waist is like a ball bearing that allows the upper and lower body to twist and rotate freely: *"Lian quan bu lian yao, zhong jiu zhi bu gao, yao wei zhongxin zhi zhou ye, yao bu huo, ze zhoushen bu lingyan"* (練拳不練腰, 終久藝不高, 腰為中心之軸也, 腰不活, 則周身不靈焉).

Today's exercises will tone and strengthen the stomach and abdominal muscles of your waist. Day by day, you'll feel these little-used muscles firming up.

WAIST STRETCH
(Hui Yao)

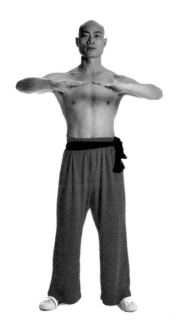 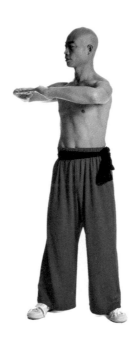 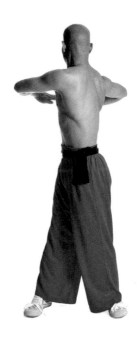

Hui Yao (pronounced *hoy yow*) is a waist stretch. Stand straight and relaxed, fully extended, with your feet comfortably apart. Hold your arms out in front of your chest, with your elbows bent so that your fingertips are pointing at each other, palms facing down.

Now twist your torso to the right, and make sure to follow with your head. Keep your lower body, from the hips down, facing forward so that you're turning only your upper body. This gives the waist and abdominal muscles a good, twisting stretch.

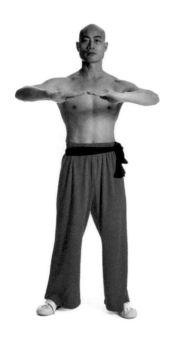
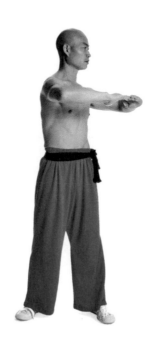
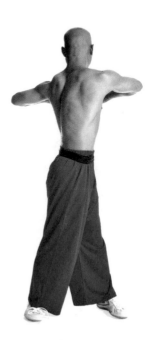

After twisting to the right, twist to the left, then to the right, then to the left, and so on. Be mindful of keeping your feet firmly planted, like the roots of a tree. Do it with some speed, and put some chi into it! Repeat for a count of 10.

WAIST ROTATION
(Rin Yao)

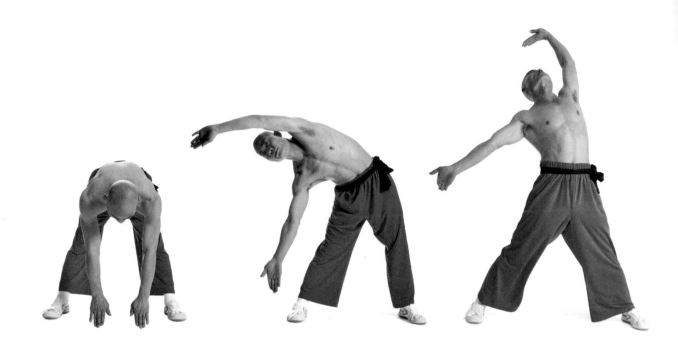

Rin Yao (pronounced *rin yow*) is a waist rotation with arms.

With your feet spread apart wider than your shoulders, bend forward at the waist as far as you can comfortably go. Ideally, you can bend far enough so that you're facing the ground. Let your arms hang in front of you, fingers pointing at the ground.

Now imagine that you're giving a big, wide circular wave to the world. Lead with your left arm, crossing in front of the right as you rotate it *counterclockwise*, and follow with your right arm. When you begin to rotate your left arm, lean your body back, arching your back so far that you are looking behind you. Keep rotating your arms and body in a full, wide counterclockwise circle until you are back where you started, bent forward at the waist. Without a

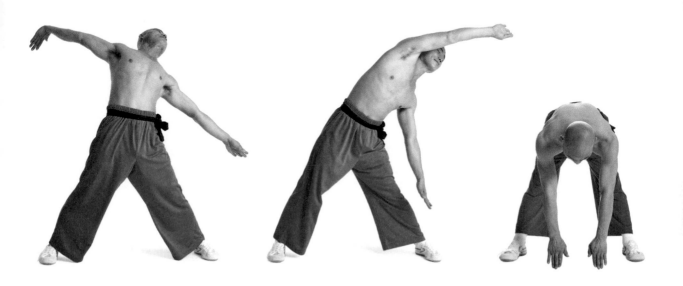

pause, continue rotating your arms and body, moving in big, smooth circles. Do it for a count of 10. Keep your knees loose and relaxed, without actually bending them.

Repeat 10 times in the opposite direction, leading with your right arm, crossing in front of your left as you rotate it *clockwise*, followed by the left arm. Rotate both arms in full, wide clockwise circles, following with your body.

It might make you feel a little dizzy the first time you try it, but this is a great exercise. You'll feel it stretching and toning your abdominals. You'll feel it stretching and relaxing your lower spine. When you do it with some chi and fully extended, you'll even feel it stretching and working the muscles in your thighs. Day by day, you'll get better at it.

Meditation

*My heart is in harmony with my mind. My mind is in harmony
with my chi. My chi is in harmony with my power.*
Xin yu yi he, yi yu qi he, qi yu li he (心與意和, 意與氣和, 氣與力和).

There are intrinsic harmonies between certain parts of the body. Your hands are in harmony with your feet. Your elbows are in harmony with your knees. And your shoulders are in harmony with your hips. As you continue to train the warrior's way, you will begin to find all the muscles and joints in your body working in harmony, giving you a strength and endurance you've probably never felt before. The Shaolin Workout trains your body from head to toe. No single muscle or limb can be anywhere near as strong as when all your muscles work together.

These physical harmonies reflect spiritual and mental harmonies: Your heart is in harmony with your mind. Your mind is in harmony with your chi. Your chi is in harmony with your power.

These are inseparable relationships. You can't separate your heart from your mind, or your mind from your body. The physical and the mental are linked. When your body is weak and tired, so is your mind. When your body falls asleep, your mind stops working, too. And by the same token, if you exhaust your mind, your body will be exhausted, too. If you're thinking and worrying so much at night that you can't rest, the next day your body will have no chi. You'll be doing your workout Sleeping Style!

That is why we relax both our bodies and our minds. We want flexible minds in flexible bodies.

If you find yourself getting stressed-out today—at your desk at work, in a long line at the supermarket, wherever it is—take a moment to relax. If your mind is stressed, your body tenses. You feel the muscles in your neck tighten, and your shoulders hunching. Your chest constricts, and you can't breathe right. You can give yourself a headache or stomachache.

When you're tense, you can't celebrate your beautiful life. Loosen up. Relax your body and your mind. Stand up from your desk and do your neck stretches and shoulder rotations. Or do them standing right there in that supermarket line. Who cares if other people are watching? Untense those muscles, and you'll relieve some of the mental stress as well. It's not magic or mumbo jumbo. It's your body and mind working in harmony. And now that you're relaxed, you'll see how much easier it is to get through the task at hand. A relaxed mind in a relaxed body allows the chi to flow and releases your power.

Try it today. You'll see.

"AMITUOFO! AMITUOFO! AMITUOFO!"

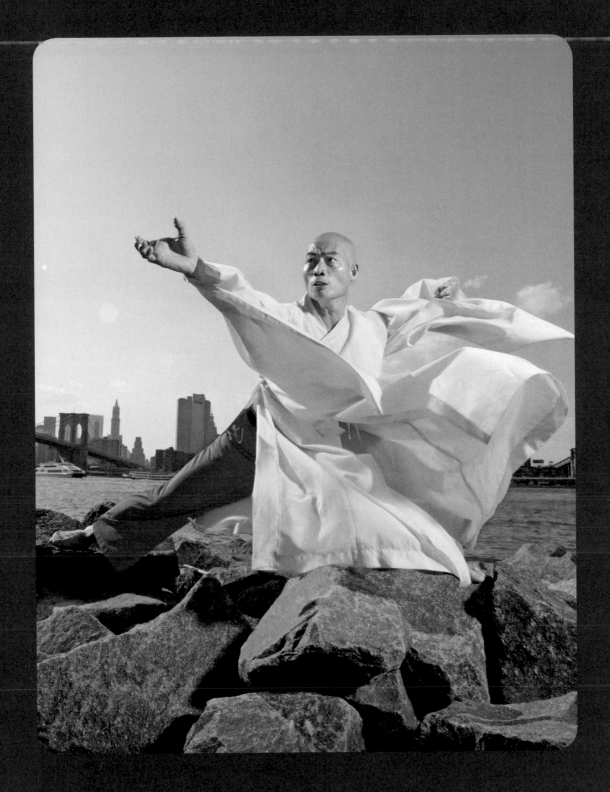

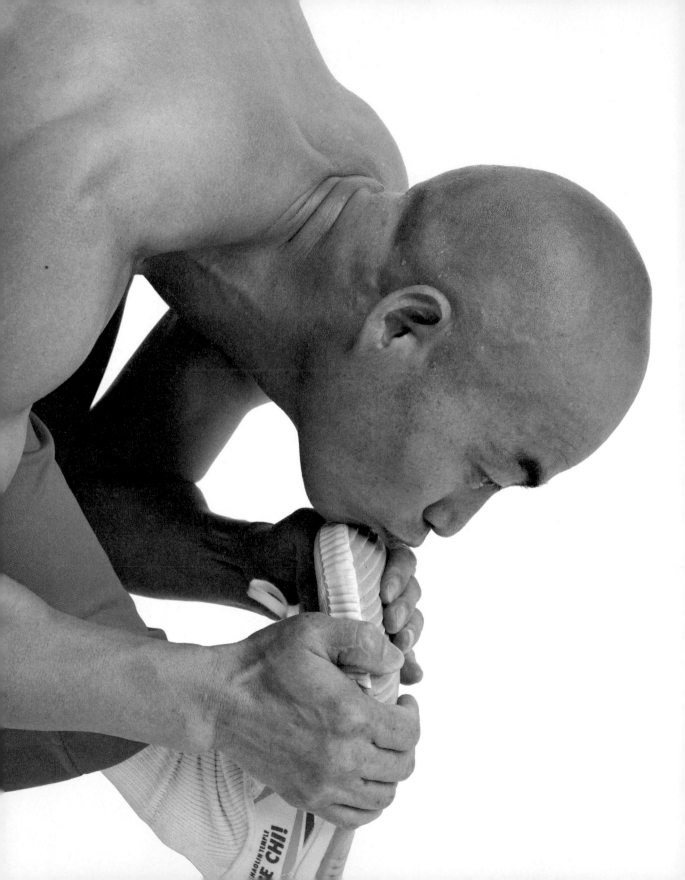

SESSION 5
Legs

"AMITUOFO!"
"AMITUOFO!"
"AMITUOFO!"

Begin by doing the previous 13 exercises.

Recall just a few days ago, when the first few exercises seemed difficult? Now you're breezing through them. That's the beauty of practice and training. Your body is loosening up and toning up every day. Your muscles are enjoying the work and asking for more.

Today we start working the legs. The kung fu warrior is an impeccably coordinated machine, from the crown of his head to the tips of his fingers and toes. The legs are an extremely important element. A tiger's claws and teeth would be useless to him if he did not have powerful legs to give him his explosive attack speed. The kung fu warrior kicks with her legs to strike farther than she can with her arms. In kung fu they say that the hands open the door for the legs: *"Shou shi liang shan men quan ping jiao da ren"* (手是兩扇門, 全憑腳打人).

As you continue to train the warrior's way, you'll soon feel the difference as your thighs and buttocks firm up, your hamstrings become more elastic and supple, and you develop a powerful coordination from your ankles and knees to your hips and lower spine.

FORWARD EXTENDED LEG STRETCH

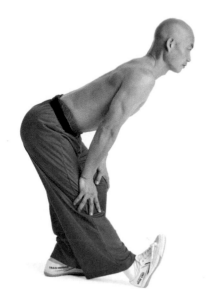

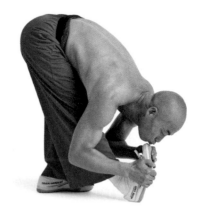

You can begin with either leg. For this example, begin with the right leg.

Stand straight and relaxed, fully extended, with your feet close together. Make sure your toes are pointing straight forward. Place your right heel in front of you, and bend your left leg. Keep your right leg straight, knee locked, and flex your foot so that your toes are pointing to the sky, or farther if you comfortably can.

Lean forward, place your palms just above the knees, and press down. Don't hunch forward or curl your back, and don't lean to one side. Keep your body and legs fully extended, your chest forward, your back straight, your head and chin up.

Push down and bounce with your whole body. Feel the bounce working your legs and buttocks. Bounce in quick pulses, 20 times (*not* 10 times for this exercise). Count to 10; then count to 10 again.

When you have completed 20 stretches of the right leg, stand, relax, and then do the left leg. Repeat 20 times.

Beautiful! With practice, you will be able to extend this position farther as your muscles learn to enjoy stretching a little more every day, becoming suppler and stronger. Sifu can squat so low and bend so far forward doing this stretch that he can kiss the toes of his extended foot, and even touch his toes with his chin. That's your goal!

Note: If you are really finding it impossible at first to keep your balance while doing this exercise, there's an alternative version you can try until you get the hang of it. In this version you can use a wall, a tree, or a fence for support. You can do it with your foot against a curb as you're waiting for a bus. Stand facing the wall so that when you extend your leg, the sole of your foot is pressed flat against it. As you go into your squat and lean forward, you can place your fingertips or palms against the wall for extra support. Do the pulses 20 times. Switch legs and do 20 more pulses.

SIDE EXTENDED LEG STRETCH

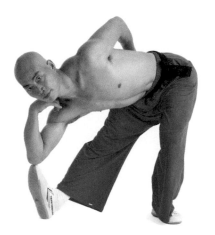 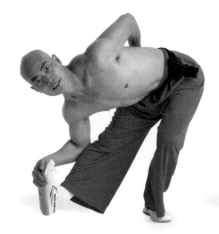 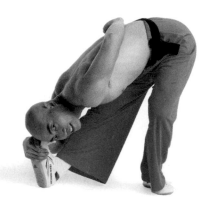

This is similar to the forward extended leg stretch. Stand straight and relaxed, fully extended, feet comfortably apart. For this example, begin with the right leg. Instead of extending it in front of you, extend it to the side, perpendicular to your body. Really stretch the leg. Keep the right knee locked. Rest your right foot on its heel and flex that foot, reaching for the sky with your toes, or farther if you can. Be mindful of keeping the left foot firmly planted.

Bend your left knee and lower your body toward the ground as you did in the previous exercise. But instead of leaning forward, extend your body sideways, over your extended right leg. Keep your chest aimed forward, your body fully extended. Placing your left arm behind your back helps to keep your body pointed forward. Extend your body as far and low as you comfortably can toward your right leg.

Bounce your upper body toward your extended leg in quick pulses. Keep the right leg and foot fully extended. Feel the stretch from your toes all the way up your back to your head. Repeat 20 times.

Rest a second. Do the left leg, 20 pulses.

Outstanding! As you continue your Shaolin Workout training, every day you'll find you're able to extend a little farther, stretching lower and lower, until you can touch your knee with your elbow, then grab your foot in your hand, then touch your toes with your head. Absolutely you will, if you train harder.

Meditation

Everyone is handsome. Everyone is beautiful.

We express ourselves through our bodies. You can see it just in a few minutes of observing people walk by on the street. If a person is depressed, lacks self-confidence, doesn't feel her own beauty, you can see it in her body and posture. She scuttles by with her shoulders hunched like she's hiding. Her head is down, her eyes fixed on the ground at her feet, hiding her face, not meeting the world eye to eye.

Then you see someone stroll by with great posture, whose back is straight, chest out, shoulders square, head up, facing the world. On Manhattan's crowded sidewalks, you can spot Sifu approaching from blocks away. He's not taller than everyone else; he just strides with such a confident, relaxed, heads-up gait that he stands out. That's someone with the self-confidence to meet the world and its challenges eye to eye. That's someone who knows he is handsome or she is beautiful. Someone who feels good inside and expresses it through his or her body.

If you're negative and lack self-confidence, other people can smell it on you like an old fish. If you're positive and self-confident, other people can smell it like a blossoming flower. Positive people will be attracted to you.

Today, remind yourself that you're beautiful. You're handsome. The Shaolin Workout helps you *express* that beauty. Don't be afraid to let your inner beauty shine out through your body. Stand up straight and proud. Square your shoulders. Lift your head. Meet the world face-to-face and eye to eye, with confidence. Remember that your body and mind are in harmony. When your body is feeling and looking good, it has a powerful positive effect on your mental state and attitude. When your mind is clear, your attitude positive, you express that with your body. The physical and the mental are inseparable, just like the body and the head.

Life is so beautiful, and so short. Appreciate your life. Celebrate your life. Live positively, seriously, honestly, understanding and expressing 100 percent of your true beauty, every moment.

"AMITUOFO! AMITUOFO! AMITUOFO!"

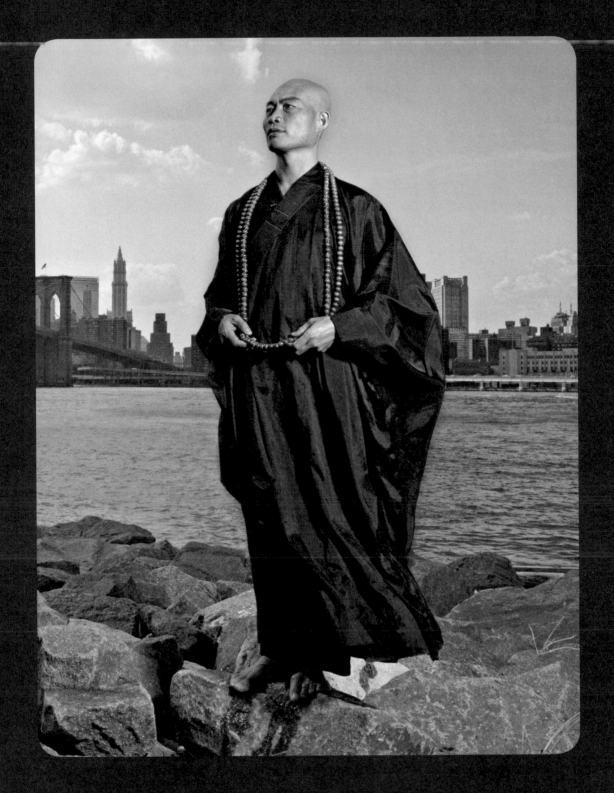

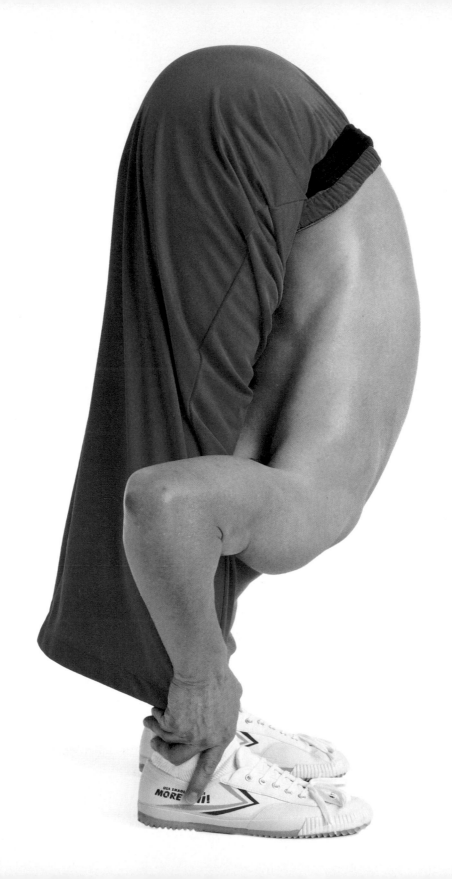

SESSION 6
Upper Body and Lower Back

"AMITUOFO!"

"AMITUOFO!"

"AMITUOFO!"

Begin by doing the previous 15 exercises.

We spend so much time sitting around at home, in the car, at work, day after day, year after year. It puts terrible pressure on the lower spine and the lower-back muscles. We're built to stand upright, with our backs stretched comfortably and our spines gently curving inward. Instead, we sit, with our spines curled outward and our backs hunched. It's no wonder so many of us experience lower-back problems, not to mention problems in the hips, knees, and ankles.

The next set of exercises will do wonders to stretch your upper body and simultaneously loosen up your lower back, stretch out those underused muscles, make you limber and flexible again like you were as a child. They may seem hard at first, because your muscles are stiff, your spine rusty, like an old screw stuck in a hole. But day by day, through dedicated repetition, you will feel the difference. And you'll look so beautiful, so handsome.

UPPER-BODY SIDE STRETCH

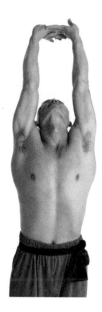

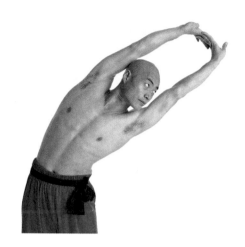

In Chinese, this exercise is called Shuag Shou Tuo Tian Shi (雙手托天式): "Two Hands Holding the Sky." Stand straight and relaxed, fully extended, with your feet close together. Lace your fingers together in front of your waist, palms toward the sky.

Now lift your arms straight out and up until your hands are all the way over your head. Keep your shoulders open and your elbows straight. Rotate your wrists so that your palms are facing the sky—holding up the sky.

Stretch your arms toward the sky. Use your hands to pull yourself up, as though you could lift yourself off the ground—but keep your feet firmly planted. Keep looking up at your hands throughout this exercise. Don't go up on the balls of your feet. This is all arms and upper body pulling you toward the sky. Fully extend. Feel the stretch all the way from your wrists down through your shoulders and down your spine and sides to your feet. Doesn't that feel great?

Now stretch to the left side. Keeping your arms in their fully extended position over your head, extend your body to the left. Don't twist it—keep facing forward. Just lean from the

waist, keeping your hips and legs steady and straight. Use the muscles on your right side to keep pushing yourself farther to the left. Keep your arms fully extended as you lean. Keep going … keep going. Extend as far to the left as you comfortably can. Stand straight again, keeping your arms fully extended overhead, and repeat the stretch to the right.

Make sure to keep your chest facing forward, your body and legs fully extended. Don't twist. Be mindful not to bend your knees.

Alternate left and right, 10 times to each side. *Yi*—left and right. *Er*—left and right. *San*—left and right. *Si*—left and right …

Beautiful. Stand straight and relax. You feel a difference already in your lower back, don't you? If you sit behind a desk at work, this is a fantastic exercise to do periodically throughout the day. Just get up from your desk and do it. During a long flight or train ride, step into the aisle and stretch. Guaranteed: When you get up to leave at the end of the day or the ride, you won't feel all stiff and hunched over like you usually do.

UPPER-BODY FORWARD STRETCH

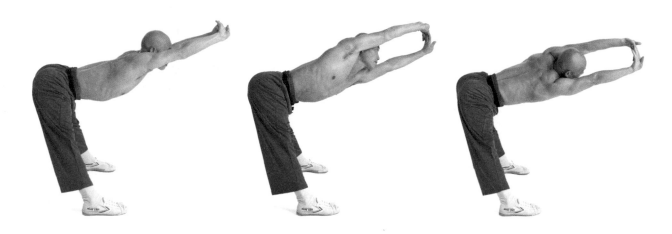

Now that you've stretched side to side, stretch forward. Stand straight and relaxed, fully extended, your feet slightly wider than your shoulders. Fully extend your legs, lock your knees, and plant your feet firmly, making your legs a firm, upside-down V shape that's your support system for the exercise.

Slowly bend forward from the hips, lowering your upper body in one smooth, slow motion. Don't bend your knees, and don't bend or curl your back. Keep your body and legs fully extended. Use your buttocks to lower your upper body from the hips. Extend your arms down, fingers pointing to the ground. Keep going until your upper body forms a straight line parallel to the ground. Lift your head and look up, straight ahead.

Lift your arms straight out in front of you from the shoulders, fingers pointing, like Superman flying. Your upper body and arms should be one long, straight line to the tips of your fingers. Lace your fingers, palms facing out, and fully extend your arms as though someone were standing in front of you, pulling you by the wrists. Use your buttock and thigh muscles to stand your ground as

your arms and back and spine stretch and extend forward. Imagine that one person is standing in front of you, pulling your wrists forward, and another is behind you, pulling your hips back. Feel it opening up your shoulders, stretching your spine, your buttocks, your hamstrings, all the way down to your feet. Count to 10.

Now, as long as you're down there, add one more element. Hold the position, arms stretched, palms out, and twist your upper body to the left, raising your right shoulder to the sky, lowering your left shoulder toward the ground. Really stretch your right side. You'll feel it all down your side and in your legs. Hold it for a beat. Twist to the right—left shoulder to sky, right shoulder to ground. Do it 10 times. *Yi*—left. *Er*—right. *San*—left. *Si*—right . . .

You look gorgeous!

You can also practice this stretch holding on to a wall, a stretching bar, a tree, a fence, or a signpost for support. If you are training with a partner, you can practice this stretch facing each other, linking your arms.

LOWER-BACK FORWARD STRETCH

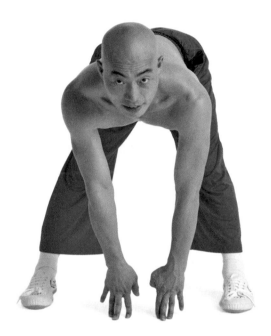 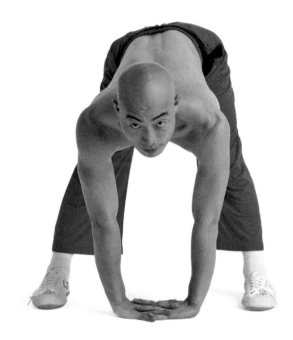

This exercise flows straight from the previous two exercises. In the upper-body side stretch, you reached for the sky and stretched from side to side. In the upper-body forward stretch, you bent forward at the waist and reached forward. Now you'll bend forward and touch the ground.

Stand straight and relaxed, fully extended, your feet slightly wider than your shoulders. Lock your knees

to make your legs that strong V-shaped support system.

Bend forward at the waist and lower your upper body, the way you did in the upper-body forward stretch. Keep your legs extended and your knees locked. Keep your back straight and fully extended. Don't slouch or curl your back. Hold your arms straight down, fingers laced, palms

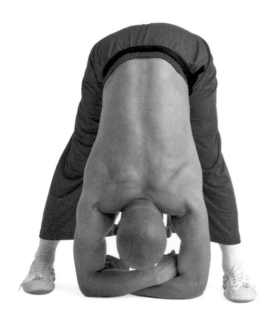
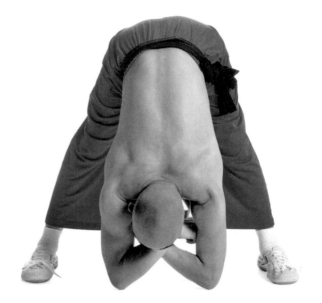

to the ground. Your goal is to touch the ground with your palms—without bending your knees. If you can't get there at first, try pulsing or bouncing your body from the hips, pushing yourself a little farther down with each bounce.

Extend as far as you comfortably can today. Tomorrow you'll get a little lower. Try to touch the ground with your palms. Then go farther, until you can extend far enough to touch the ground with your elbows as you bounce. You'll get there. Train harder!

ANKLE GRIP

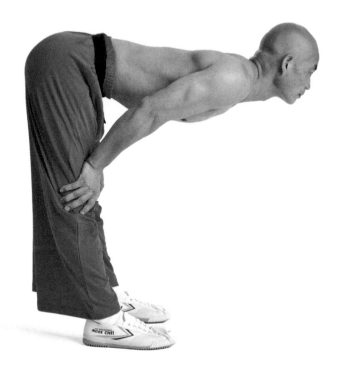

This exercise further stretches your lower back and hamstrings. It continues and flows directly from the previous exercise. Stand straight and relaxed, fully extended, with your feet comfortably apart, as wide as your shoulders. Place your hands at your sides, palms against your outer thighs.

Lock your knees and bend forward at the waist, lowering your body toward the ground, as you've been doing in the previous two exercises. As you lower your body, slide your palms down the outsides of your legs. Keep bending, and keep sliding your hands down to your knees, then down to your calves. Keep your knees locked.

Keep going until your hands can grip your ankles. When you've reached your ankles, the top of your head should be very near to touching the ground. Bounce your upper body up and down from the buttocks, like you did in the

previous exercise. Do it for a 10 count. Remember to keep your feet firmly planted and your knees locked.

Stand straight again, keeping your feet at shoulder width.

Bend forward at the waist, keeping your back extended, and place your palms above your knees, with your thumbs on your inner thighs. Bounce your lower back up and down 10 times, keeping your back extended, your knees and elbows locked, and your hands above your knees. As you bounce your lower back, push against your legs with your palms, keeping your elbows locked.

Bring your feet closer together so they are a bit wider than your head. Slide your hands down your legs as you continue to lower your body. Your goal is to grip your ankles and fold yourself in half at the waist so that your head is upside-down between your ankles and you're looking behind you!

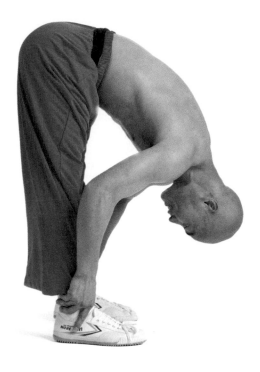
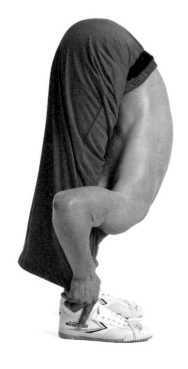

Don't cheat by bending your knees. You'd only be cheating yourself. Go as far as you comfortably can today. Tomorrow you'll be able to stretch it a bit farther, and farther the next day. Train harder! You'll love the results.

Note: Right now you may be saying, "But Sifu, I can hardly bend forward at all. My back is so stiff. I'll never touch the ground with my fingertips, let alone my elbows. I'll never be able to grip my ankles."

If you're really having a lot of trouble getting started with these exercises, there's a beginner's stretch you can practice for a few days to loosen your back up. You use a wall, a tree, a stretching bar, a fence, or a lamppost for support. Stand facing this support at a distance almost equal to the length of your extended arms plus your upper body. Plant your feet firmly at shoulder width and keep your knees locked. Lean forward from the waist and place

your palms flat against the wall higher than your head, at shoulder width. Fully extend your back. Lower your body as far as you comfortably can without moving your hands. Try bouncing your back up and down. Look up as you do this. Do it for a count of 10. You'll feel the lower back and spine loosening up right away.

Try it standing farther back and placing your palms lower on the support so that you lean your body farther and lower. Remember to keep your knees locked, your legs, back, and arms fully extended. Bounce your back up and down 10 times.

After a day or two of this, try the previous exercise again for real. You'll be surprised how much easier it is and how it flows into this exercise. Believe in yourself. Trust yourself. Have confidence in yourself.

Meditation

Dripping water bores a hole in the rock. **Di shui chuan shi** (滴水穿石).

For many people, today's stretches cannot be executed right away. You may have to practice, practice, practice, stretching, stretching, and stretching. You may feel like you'll never be able to touch the ground with your palms, or bend yourself in half at the waist.

Don't be discouraged if it takes a while. Little by little, you will improve. There is a Chinese saying—a *cheng yu*, similar to what's called a proverb in the West: "Dripping water bores a hole in the rock." There's a rock outside your house, directly under a hole in the rain gutter, where a slow, steady drip-drip-drip of droplets falls whenever it rains. A single raindrop will have no effect on that rock. But every time it rains, a succession of raindrops hits that rock at exactly the same spot. Over time—a very long time—the cumulative effect of all those raindrops will begin to wear a hole in the rock. It'll take many years, but eventually those little raindrops will bore a hole straight through the rock. One raindrop could never do that, nor 10, nor 100. But slowly, gradually, with patience and perseverance, they'll make their way through, a tiny bit at a time.

In China they also say, *"Bingdong san chi fei yi ri zhi han yan"* (冰凍三尺, 非一日之寒焉): "The ice didn't get 3 feet thick overnight." When it first goes below freezing in early winter, a thin skim of ice will form on a pond. As the weeks and months of winter pass, the ice thickens, inch by inch, until the pond is frozen solid.

That's why you practice, practice, practice. The ground may seem far away at first, but each repetition moves you a little bit closer to touching it. Your improvement may be so gradual that you don't even notice, but don't give up. Be as patient as the rain and the ice.

"AMITUOFO! AMITUOFO! AMITUOFO!"

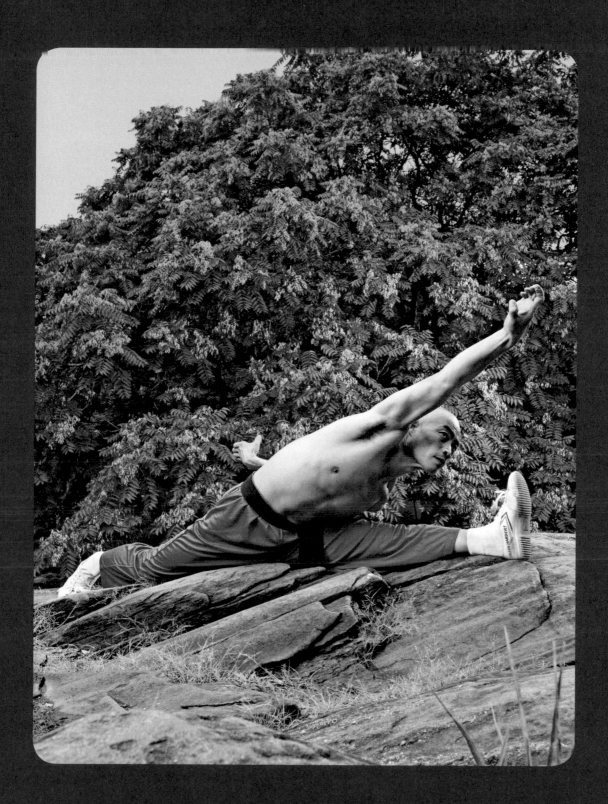

SESSION 7

Review

"AMITUOFO!"
"AMITUOFO!"
"AMITUOFO!"

Congratulations! You've completed the first week of your Shaolin Workout. You can already feel the transformation beginning, can't you?

Today, review the lessons you've learned so far. Try to do the previous 19 exercises as though the separate moves were the movements of a symphony, each flowing into the next. You may pause in between them to adopt the correct stance, but don't dawdle. Finish one movement and move on to the next, and then the next. Do them as quickly and with as much chi as you can put into them. Accelerate your counting—*Yi! Er! San! Si!* Faster! Farther! You *can* do it!

Speed is key in Chan Quan. From speed comes power. You will actually find that the faster and more energetically you do the movements, the better you will get at them. You will truly find yourself doing the exercises more easily as you speed them up. Partly that's because you're warming up your muscles more quickly, so they're more elastic, which means they can stretch farther. But it's also because the faster you do the movements, the less you'll be thinking about them. Your body will just do them, as instinctively and naturally as a tiger flashes across an open field. You will become a pure mind in a beautiful body. That is one meaning of action meditation.

Review your daily meditations today as well. They're integral to your transformation. Recommit yourself to your goal of developing a relaxed mind in a relaxed body, as graceful and poised in your attitude as in your limbs. Remind yourself of how beautiful you are. Don't let the stresses or minor disappointments of your day distract you from this wonderful project of self-discovery and self-transformation. If you find life stressing you out, stretch it out! Don't let yourself tense up and block your chi. Let it flow.

You're doing great. As you begin Part Two, cheer yourself on. More chi! Train harder!

"AMITUOFO!"
"AMITUOFO!"
"AMITUOFO!"

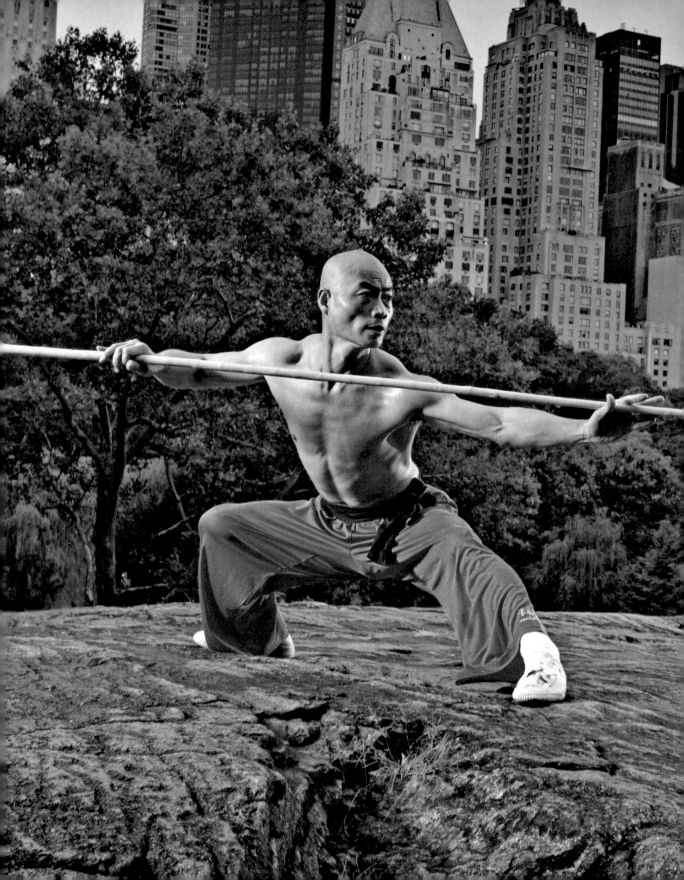

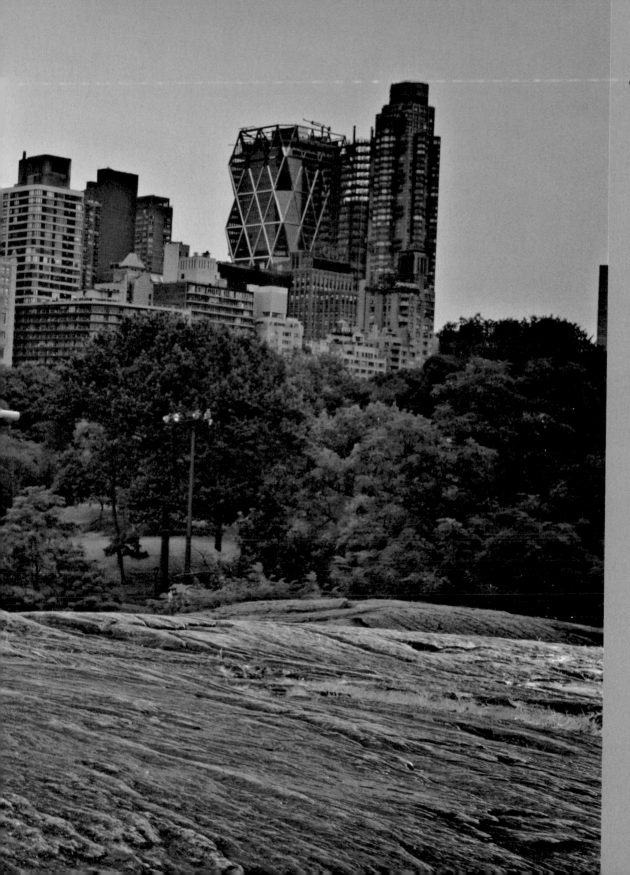

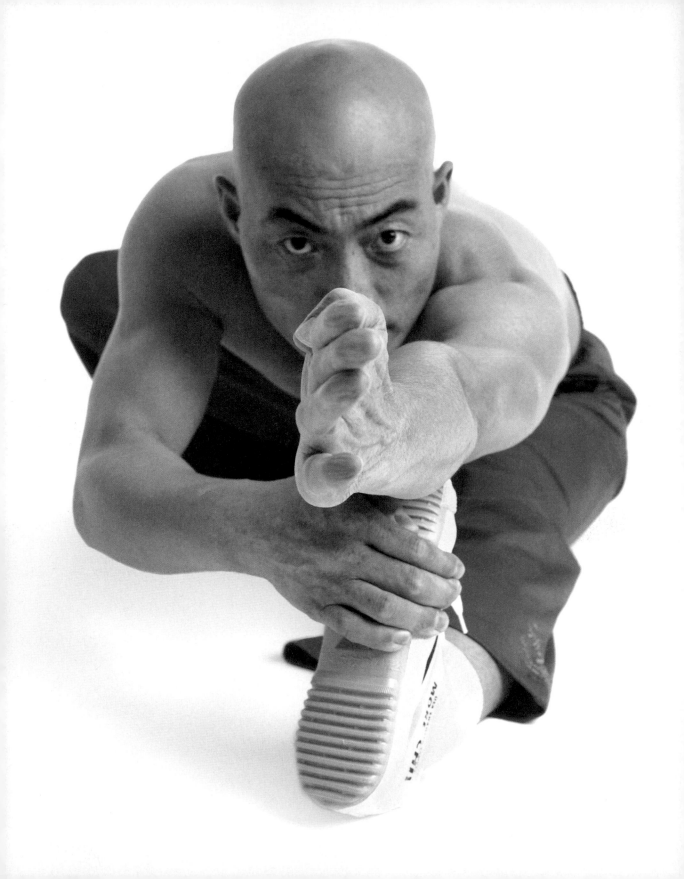

SESSION 8
Hamstrings and Hips

"AMITUOFO!"
"AMITUOFO!"
"AMITUOFO!"

Begin by doing all the previous exercises, quickly and fluidly.

GONG BU STRETCH
(Gong Bu Yatui)

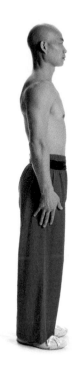
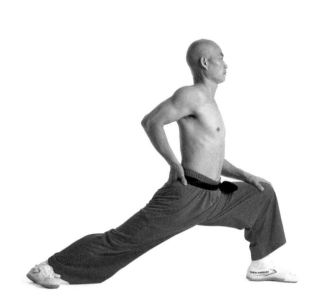

The stance called Gong Bu, which you will learn in a few days, is one of the most important fundamentals of kung fu. Today you will learn the stretch—*yatui* (pronounced *yah-twee*) is Chinese for "stretch"—on which Gong Bu is based. It strengthens your legs, buttocks, and groin.

Stand straight and relaxed, fully extended, hands at your sides.

You can begin with either leg; for this example, let's make it the left leg. Take a comfortable step forward with your left leg and plant your foot flat, toes facing straight ahead. Your right leg will be extended behind you, knee locked. Bend your left knee and squat at least until your left thigh is parallel to the ground. (If you can get even lower, go for it.) Be mindful to keep your upper body fully extended, chest

forward, shoulders square, head and chin up. Don't let your body turn outward or hunch forward. Also, maintain "a closed groin." In other words, don't let your hips splay open.

Grip your left thigh with your left hand, just above the knee. Put your right hand behind you and press the palm to the top of your right buttock. Do pulsing squats, pushing your left leg and your butt toward the ground with your hands. Bounce down and up, down and up, remembering to keep your body and back leg fully extended, and both feet firmly planted. Don't let the back foot lift up. Do 10 pulses.

Now reverse, without standing up—right leg forward, left leg fully extended behind you, and do 10 pulses.

Wow, look at you go! That's so fantastic!

HIP STRETCH

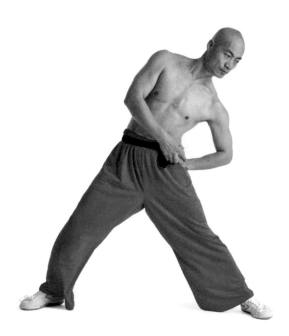 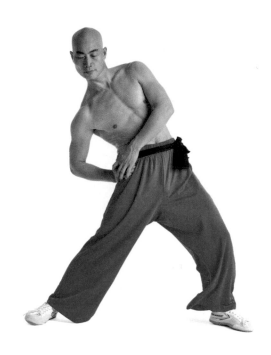

This exercise continues directly from the Gong Bu stretch. When you've completed that stretch, don't stand up; stay in position, with your right (or forward) thigh parallel to the ground, your left leg extended and locked behind you, both feet planted firm and flat on the ground. Turn your whole body 90 degrees to the left, pivoting on both feet, so that your shoulders and knees are in line with each other. Keep your right knee bent. Don't lift your feet or take a step; keep them planted firm and flat, and just pivot them so that your toes are pointing in the same direction that you're facing. Be mindful to keep your body fully extended, and your left leg fully extended as well, knee locked.

Place both hands on the left side of your waist, just above the hip bone, right hand over the left. Stretch your body to the left, using your hands to help push your hips to the right. Now pulse to the side 10 times.

Excellent!

Now reverse. Place your palms on the right side of your waist just above the hip bone, left over right, and extend your body to the right. Pulse to the side 10 times.

PU BU STRETCH
(Pu Bu Yatui)

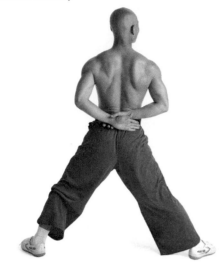

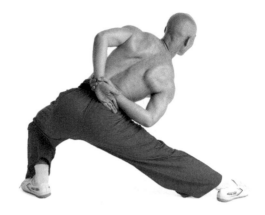

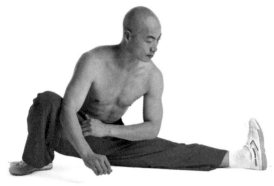

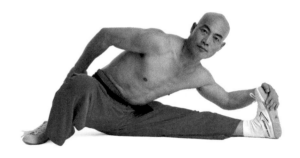

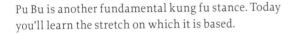

Pu Bu is another fundamental kung fu stance. Today you'll learn the stretch on which it is based.

Pu Bu Yatui *(poo-boo yah-twee)* flows directly from the hip stretch. You can begin with either side. Let's stretch the right side first.

Execute a hip stretch with the left knee bent and the right leg fully extended, knee locked. Extend your body to the right, leaning over your extended right leg; at the same time, lower your body toward the ground, crouching as low as you comfortably can. Extend your body as far as you can to the right without turning your body. Fold

yourself in half from the hip until your side is against your right leg. If you can, grip your right foot with your right hand and your left foot with your left hand, keeping both feet firmly flat and remembering to keep your right leg fully extended and your knee locked. Your goal is to extend your body to the right until you can not only grip that foot but extend your palm out past it.

Pulse down and to the side 10 times. Then hold that stretch for a count of 10. You'll feel it from your toes up your legs and all the way up your back.

Rise and switch legs without moving your feet, extending

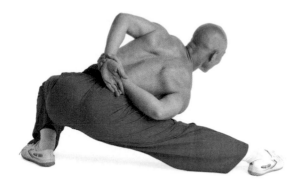

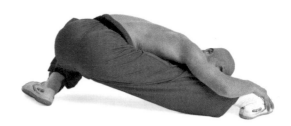

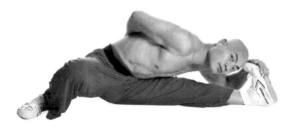

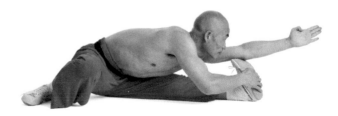

to the left this time. Pulse down and to the side 10 times; then hold it for a 10 count.

When you've held that Pu Bu Yatui to the left for a 10 count, add one more element: a half split. Lower your body all the way until your butt touches the ground. Flex your left foot so that it's on its heel, pointing your toes to the sky or, if you can, toward you. Keep your right foot planted firm and flat. Fully extend your body toward your flexed left foot. Fold yourself in half at the hip as you lean as far as you can over your extended left leg. It helps to bounce your body to the left. Your goal is to extend your body so far to the left that you can grab that foot in both hands and then touch

the toes of your left foot with your left ear, and stretch your left arm out past your toes, all the way to the elbow.

Stretch as far as you can comfortably go to the left today, and hold it for a 10 count. Then reverse, executing a half split to the right.

Note: When you're practicing Pu Bu Yatui and half splits, stretch and extend only as far as you comfortably can today. Tomorrow you'll get a little farther. Every body is unique, and we all start out at different degrees of flexibility. If you can't stretch as far as Sifu can now, with dedicated training you'll keep increasing your flexibility until you can.

Meditation

Merry Christmas! Happy New Year!

Every day, no matter what time of year it is, Sifu greets people with cheers of "Merry Christmas!" If they've been around him more than a few minutes, they smile and reply, "Happy New Year, Sifu!"

If that seems silly in the middle of July, there's a wonderful message behind it. It's Sifu's way of asking, "Why do we celebrate our beautiful lives only on specific days of the year? Why is it only our birthdays and anniversaries, Christmas and Hanukkah and New Year's? Why isn't every day a celebration?"

Why do we enjoy holidays? Because we don't have to work, we're surrounded by family, we have great meals, we laugh and play.

But why limit your happiness to just those few special days of the year? You should be that happy every day, every hour, every minute. Why limit your heart and mind?

Life is beautiful. Every day is a good day. Today it may be sunny. That's beautiful—let's go to the beach! It makes everybody happy. Yesterday it rained. That was beautiful, too! Clouds are beautiful. It's like God made a big painting in the sky. We need the rain. The world would be a lifeless desert without rain. Every living thing on the planet—the beautiful flowers, the grass, the trees, the corn, the wheat, and all the animals—needs the rain. We need water to drink and to cook with, to take our showers and baths, to use the toilet. Snow is fantastic, too. Each snowflake is unique, like a tiny sculpture, no two ever alike. How marvelous is that?

Celebrate your beautiful life every day, whatever it brings. Live today as though it were Christmas. And tomorrow? Happy New Year! Celebrate life 8 days a week and 366 days a year!

"AMITUOFO! AMITUOFO! AMITUOFO!"

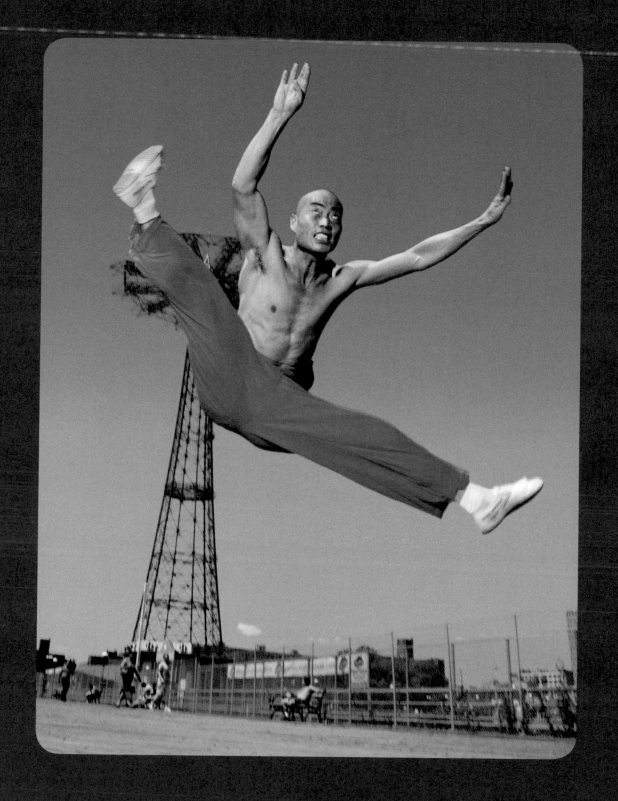

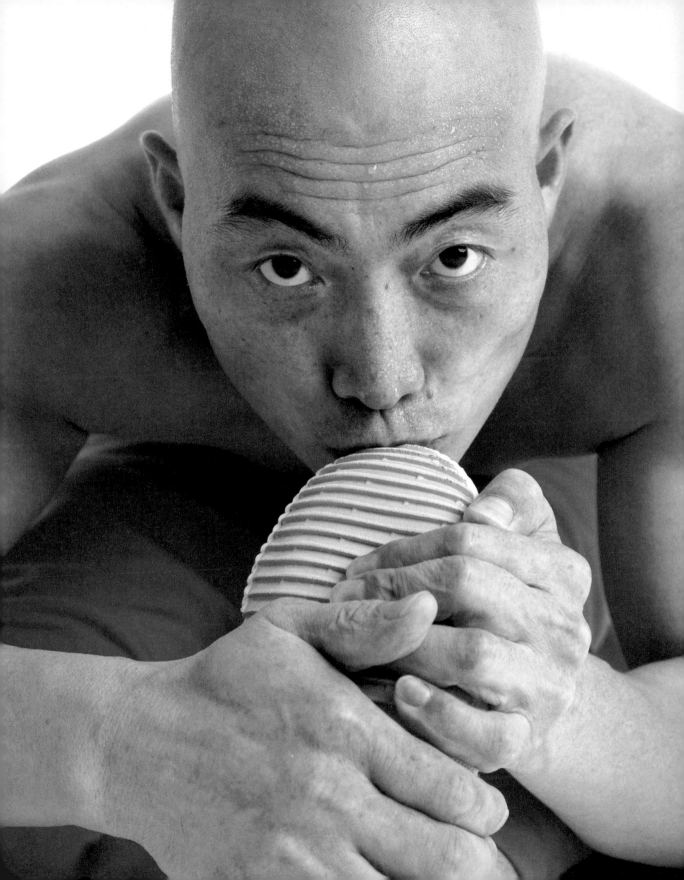

SESSION 9

Hips, Knees, and
Warm-Down Stretches

"AMITUOFO!"
"AMITUOFO!"
"AMITUOFO!"

Begin by doing all the previous exercises.

How far can you stretch your back today? How close are you to touching the ground when you do the lower-back forward stretch? Very good! More chi! Train harder!

Today, because you've been training so hard, treat yourself to some easier stretches.

HIP ROTATION

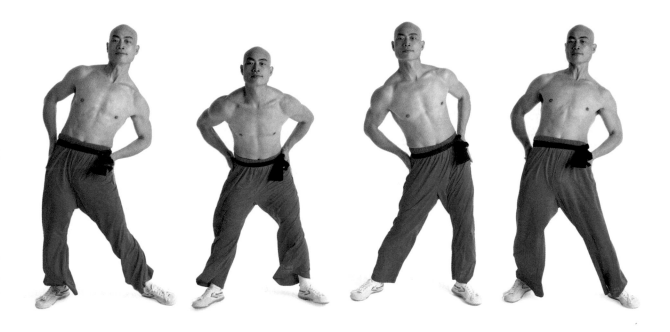

Stand straight and relaxed, fully extended, with your feet spread slightly wider than shoulder width, your toes pointing straight forward.

Reach behind you and place your palms on your buttocks. Rotate your hips in a circle. Make the circle as big and wide as you can. Don't bend your knees—keep your legs fully extended as your hips circle above them. Also keep your feet firmly planted on the ground. And keep your body facing forward and fully extended as your hips make their circles under it.

Make 10 big, wide, fully extended circles in one direction; then reverse, doing 10 in the other direction.

Awesome!

KNEE ROTATION

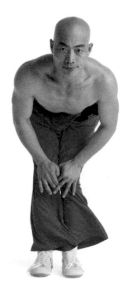 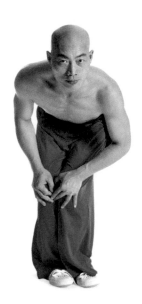 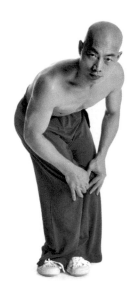 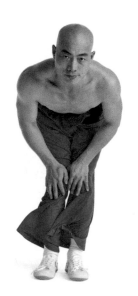

Stand straight and relaxed, fully extended, your legs closed, your feet close together and pointed forward.

Now reach down and grab your knees. Keep your knees relaxed and bent. Now, keeping your legs together and your feet firmly planted on the ground, rotate your knees in a circle. Make it as wide as you can. Extend.

Do it 10 times in one direction and then 10 times in the other direction.

Gorgeous! Now learn two seated warm-down stretches that feel fantastic at the end of a long, strenuous workout—or a long day at the office, or a long flight....

SEATED HAMSTRING STRETCH

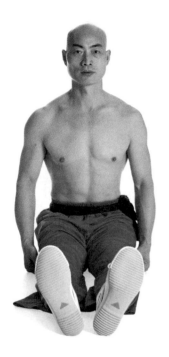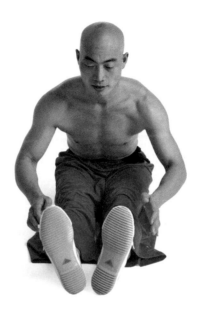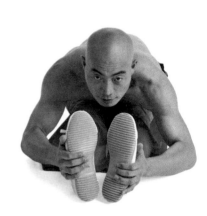

Sit on the ground. Extend your legs out straight in front of you, with a few inches of space between them. Lock your knees. Flex your feet so your toes are pointed toward you. Fully extend your feet and legs. You'll know when your legs and feet are at full extension because your heels will naturally lift off the ground while the backs of your thighs are pressed flat against it. Also fully extend your back. Reach for the sky with the top of your head.

Do not slouch, slump, or curl your spine at any point in this stretch.

Now you'll fold yourself in half from the hips. Slowly lean forward over your legs, sliding your hands down the outside of your legs as you lower yourself. Remember, do not curl or hunch your back—keep it straight and fully extended. Don't bend your knees, either. Your first goal is

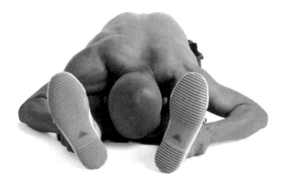 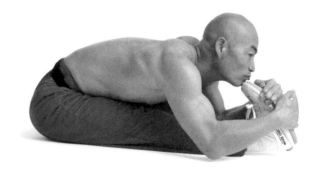

to bend yourself in half at the waist until your hands grip your feet and you can kiss the ground between your calves. When you can stretch that far comfortably, keep going. Your ultimate goal is to extend until you can kiss your toes. Show them how much you appreciate them for carrying you around all day! Also touch them with your chin.

Hold that position for a moment, feeling it stretch your lower spine and the backs of your thighs. Then gradually lift yourself back up to the seated position.

Don't worry if you can't kiss your toes today. With daily practice, you will. And your lower back and hamstrings will bless you for it.

CROSSED SEATED STRETCHES

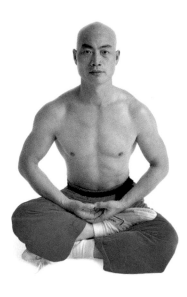

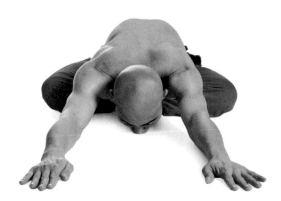

Sit on the ground with your knees bent and your right leg fully on top of the left, right foot on left thigh in the half lotus position. Your back should be straight and fully extended. Lean forward over your legs, without letting your back curl. Keep leaning until you can slide the palms of your hands across the ground and kiss the ground. Don't hunker or hunch. Keep your back fully extended and arched as you fold yourself to the ground. Hold that position for a moment; then slowly rise back up to the seated position.

Fold yourself forward again, but this time curl your back and extend until the top of your head touches the ground. Hold this position for a moment.

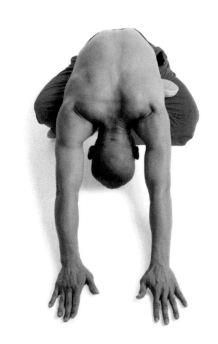

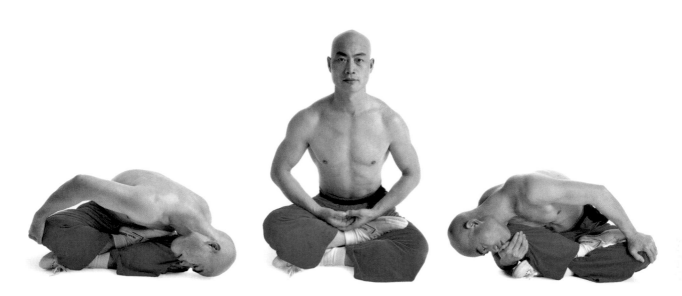

Rise to a sitting position again and relax for a moment. Now stretch from side to side as well. Lean your upper body as far as you can over your left side and hold that position for a moment. Kiss your knee and toes while you're there, to show them your apprecia-tion. Rise, and repeat the lean to the right, kissing that knee and toes.

Sit up and relax for a moment. The stretch you just performed is called Dan Pan.

(continued)

CROSSED SEATED STRETCHES (cont.)

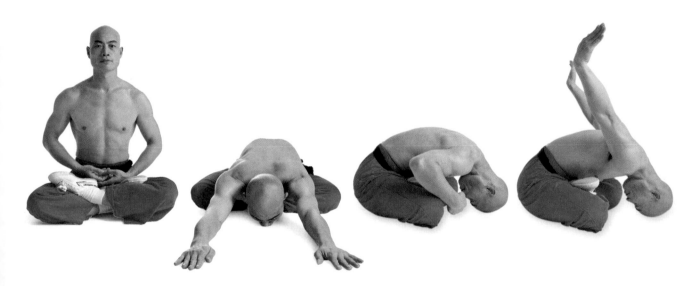

Now you're going to perform the stretch called
Son Pan. Remain sitting with your right foot on your left
thigh, and pull up your left foot so that it is on your right
thigh in the full lotus position. Lean forward, folding
yourself in half from the waist, keeping your back
arched and fully extended. Slide your hands across the
ground and continue to lower yourself until you can kiss
the ground.

Sit up and relax.

Fold yourself in half at the waist again, curling your
back this time until the top of your head touches
the ground. While you're down there, extend your
arms behind your back and as high as you can
toward the sky, with the wrists bent so the palms
face forward.

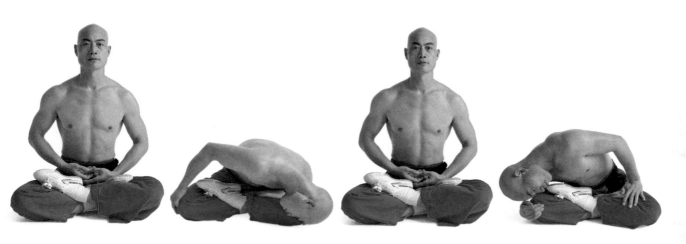

Hold for a moment; then sit up and relax. Lean your body to the left until you can kiss that knee. Then to the right, kissing that knee. Sit up and relax.

Doesn't your lower back feel great when you're done? You'll feel yourself standing, walking, and sitting more comfortably all day.

Meditation

Flatten your heart. Pingchang xin (平常心).

China is blessed with many mountain ranges. The five most famous and revered in Buddhist tradition are Mount Tai to the east, Mount Hua to the west, Mount Heng to the north, another Mount Heng to the south, and Mount Song in the center, in Henan Province. The Song mountain range is where Shaolin Temple is located.

There are 72 smaller mountains in the Song range. In Shaolin tradition, those 72 mountains are equally divided into 36 yin and 36 yang—or 36 plus and 36 minus. The yin and the yang balance and cancel each other out. There is no plus, and no minus.

This reflects the universal balance that is the goal of Chan Buddhism. No birth, no death. No suffering, no desire. No distractions. We acknowledge this when we chant "AMITUOFO!" three times before a session and three times after. They balance each other out. They cancel each other out. No plus, no minus.

In Chan Buddhism, there is a saying: "Flatten your heart." This does not mean that you should act like a robot, with no emotions. But it does mean that you should not get distracted by the emotional highs and lows life throws at you. Mastering your life includes mastering your emotions. Think about how often your emotions are reactions to other people or to external forces you can't control. When you react wildly, you are giving up mastery of your life to somebody or something else. If someone is rude or insulting to you, for instance, you might be depressed for the rest of the day. That's a day you wasted. If you miss your bus and are late for work, you might be in a bad mood all day. That's also a day you wasted—not just for yourself but for everyone else whom *you* distracted with your foul mood.

To flatten your heart means not to let those external forces yank you around and distract you from your goal of polishing and perfecting your life. It means understanding that the person who makes you angry or sad isn't the one who ruins your day—*you* ruin your day by the way you react. It means to stay relaxed and balanced in mind, heart, and body. It's a tremendous waste of chi to go jumping from high highs to low lows, from really good days to really bad ones. Every day is a gift. When you break up with someone, it feels like the saddest day of your life. Then you fall in love again, and you feel like exploding with joy. That's life. It's full of sorrow and joy, highs and lows. The trick is not to let it throw you out of balance but to live each day as it comes, happy to be alive.

Keep it simple. Flatten your heart. Be mindful of the beautiful gift your life is at *this* moment.

"AMITUOFO! AMITUOFO! AMITUOFO!"

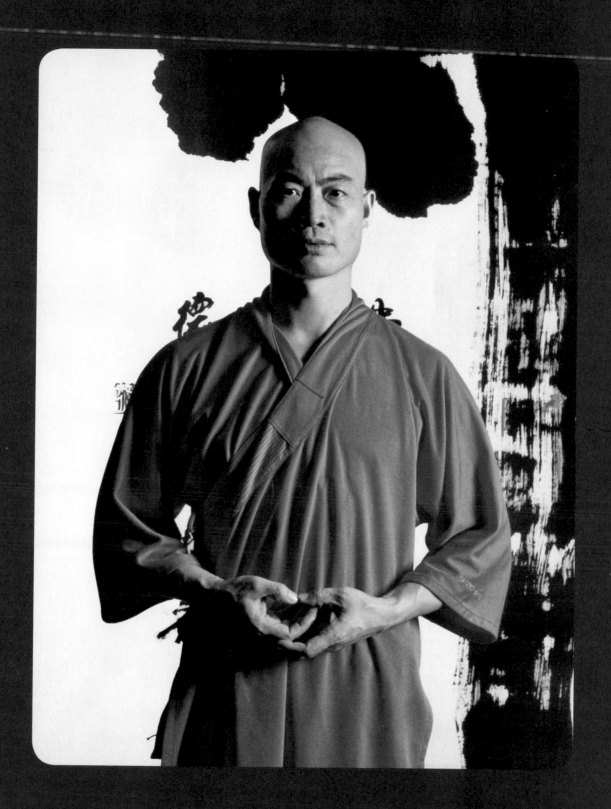

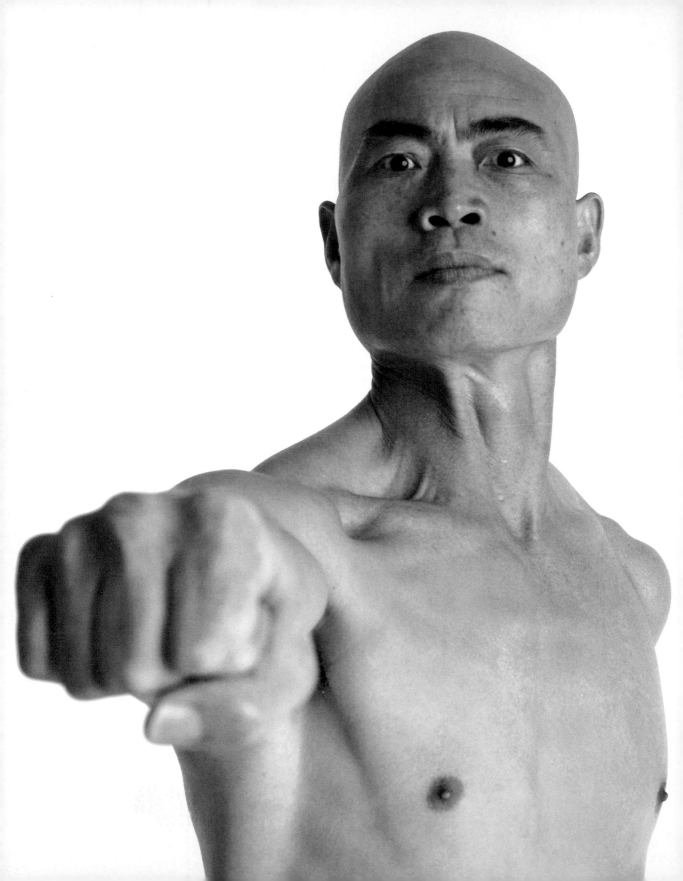

Pushing Palm Strike
Fist Punch

"AMITUOFO!"
"AMITUOFO!"
"AMITUOFO!"

Begin by practicing the previous 26 exercises.

Still falling on your behind trying to do those Pu Bu splits? Don't be embarrassed. You've only been doing them for a few days. It can take days or weeks to fully master the harder stretches. Don't give up. Think of the feeling of pride when you have them all down pat. You've learned them all. Now it's a matter of practicing and perfecting.

So let's move on to some fun stuff—the basic kung fu strikes, stances, and kicks.

Please remember as you are learning these wonderful strikes and kicks that you are *not* "learning how to fight." If you ever did get into a real fight, no move you're learning here would be of any use. You're practicing kung fu to learn intrinsic physical and spiritual harmonies; to enhance your reflexes and balance, your speed and power; to develop self-respect and self-confidence. The true kung fu warrior doesn't go looking for fights; he spreads peace and love by fully expressing the beauty of all life.

PUSHING PALM STRIKE
(Tui Zhang)

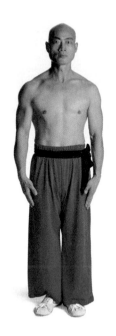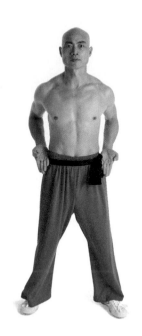

Tui Zhang (pronounced *twee jang*) is incorporated into many kung fu moves, so learning it correctly now will be of great help to you as you progress through the program.

Stand straight and relaxed, feet together, hands at sides. Now learn how to quickly assume the "ready" position, doing it smartly, like a soldier snapping to attention. In Chinese, "Ready!" is *"Yu bei!"* (pronounced *yoo bay*). Call it out to yourself when you snap into position. Then, when you strike, call out *"Zou!"* (pronounced *tzo*). It means "Go!"

Yu bei! Quickly spread your feet to a comfortable distance, slightly more than shoulder width, and, with your arms close to your body, rapidly bend your elbows straight back and slide your hands up to your waist, with your palms flat and facing the sky, fingers pointing straight ahead of you. Do it smartly, with snap.

The edges of your palms should be on your waist. Curl your thumbs in tight over your palms. This is to protect your thumbs. If you were actually striking an object (or a person) and your thumbs were hanging out, they could get bent backward painfully, or even broken. Curl those thumbs in tight and hold them there. Think of your hand as the blade of a knife, all one solid piece of steel. In Chinese they say *"Wu zhi pin long"* (五指拼攏)—"Five fingers together as one."

Now for the strike itself. To learn it, we'll break it down into a series of separate movements and then put them all together in sequence.

You can begin with either hand. For this example, let's make it the right hand.

Zou! In one smooth, quick motion, strike your right arm straight out in front of you at shoulder height. Fully extend the arm. Your wrist should bend so that your fingers are pointing toward the sky and the outer edge of your palm is pointing straight ahead. Remember to keep that thumb curled in tight. Don't move your feet. Keep them solid and flat on the ground. Your shoulder will turn slightly to follow your arm as it strikes, but don't overturn or overtwist your body. Remember, as always, to keep your body fully extended, chest out, head and chin high. Let's call this hand position 1.

Without moving any other part of your body, turn your palm so that it is facing you, and the tips of your fingers are pointing left at a 90-degree angle. This is hand position 2.

Got that? Now put 1 and 2 together into one fluid movement. With your right arm, strike, and turn your palm to hand position 2. Try it a few times until you've got the hang of it.

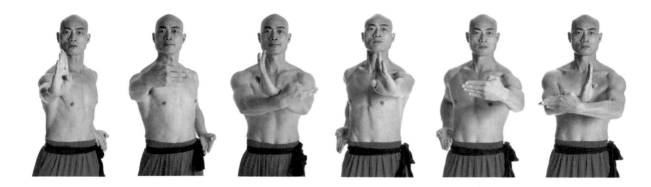

Add the left arm. First, do steps 1 and 2 with the right hand: With the right arm, strike, and turn your right palm to position 2. As you are turning your right palm, begin to strike with your left hand, crossing behind your right wrist as it strikes forward.

As your left arm is reaching full extension, simultaneously lower your right arm to its starting position. Think of a monk at Shaolin Temple in his robes with the flowing sleeves. Imagine that with his left hand he's lighting incense on the altar. As he reaches with that hand, he uses his right hand to brush his left sleeve down his arm.

When the full move is completed, your left arm should be straight out in front of you, with the edge of your palm forward, in hand position 1. Your right arm has slid back to its starting position, palm up, the edge of your palm against your waist. This is called chambering your palm.

Understand? Now put it all together into a smooth sequence of moves. Practice it slowly at first, as a set of distinct arm and hand positions. Right arm to hand position 1. Right hand to position 2. Left hand comes up behind the right. Left hand strikes as right arm slides back to the waist. As left hand turns to position 2, right arm is beginning to strike. Right hand strikes, as left arm slides back to waist . . . and so on.

Do it 20 times—two counts of 10—speeding it up as your arms learn the sequence. Do it all as one smooth concert of moves for your arms. Your two arms should be constantly alternating, one extending out and striking at the exact same time as the other slides back to your waist. They balance each other out—no yin, no yang, no plus, no minus. Right, left, right, left. *Yi, er, san, si* . . .

As you learn to speed up the movement, strike with real snap. Imagine that your arms are rubber bands, snapping out and back very quickly, extending and retracting with the same speed. You know how much a rubber band hurts when you snap one against your skin? The rubber band itself is just a thin little bit of elastic. But when you stretch and snap it—ow! Think of your strikes like that. Snap! Pow!

You'll find that the smoother and faster you strike, the less you have to think about it. And the less you think about it, the more it becomes completely instinctive and natural. Just like life—the more relaxed you are, the more comfortable, the more natural, the more power you can express. Don't think—just do it!

(continued)

PUSHING PALM STRIKE (cont.)

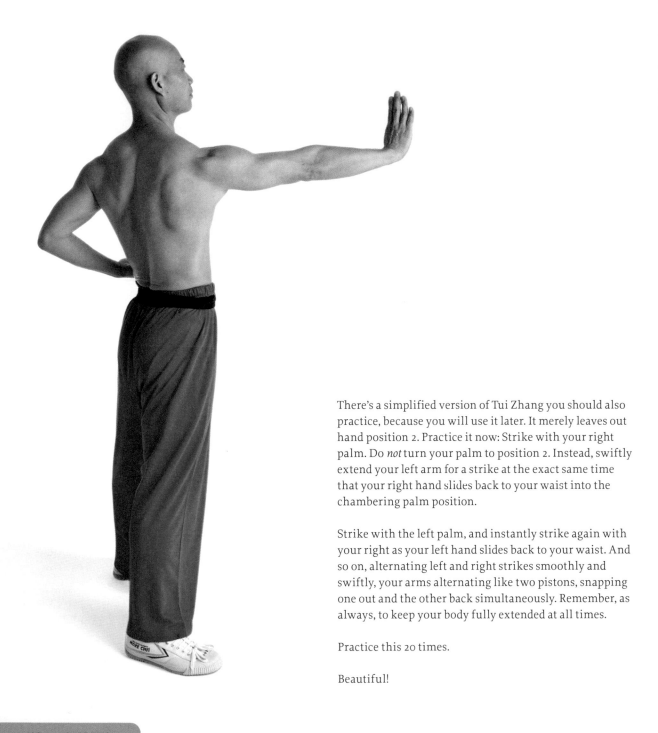

There's a simplified version of Tui Zhang you should also practice, because you will use it later. It merely leaves out hand position 2. Practice it now: Strike with your right palm. Do *not* turn your palm to position 2. Instead, swiftly extend your left arm for a strike at the exact same time that your right hand slides back to your waist into the chambering palm position.

Strike with the left palm, and instantly strike again with your right as your left hand slides back to your waist. And so on, alternating left and right strikes smoothly and swiftly, your arms alternating like two pistons, snapping one out and the other back simultaneously. Remember, as always, to keep your body fully extended at all times.

Practice this 20 times.

Beautiful!

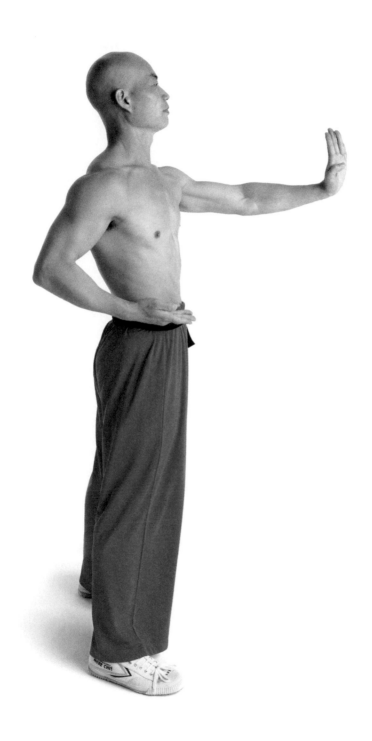

FIST PUNCH
(Chong Quan)

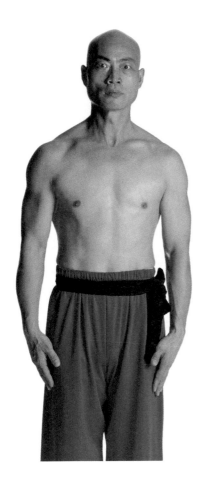 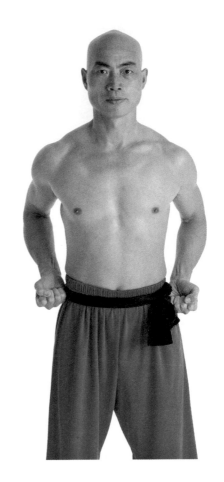

Stand straight and relaxed, feet close together, arms at sides.

Yu bei! Just as you did at the start of the palm strike, quickly spread your feet to slightly more than shoulder width, smartly bend your elbows back, and slide your hands up to your waist, palms toward the sky. But instead of having your palms flat, this time curl your fingers to make fists. In Chinese they say of this fist-making action,

"*Wo quan ru juan pian*" (握拳如捲胼). It means that it's like the rolling action of two hands twisting strands into a rope. From now on, this will be referred to as "chambering" your fists. This is the starting position for the fist punch, Chong Quan (pronounced *chong chwan*).

You can begin by striking with either fist. For this example, let's make it the right fist.

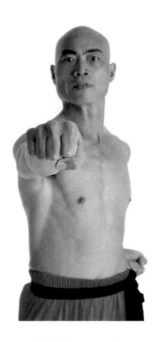
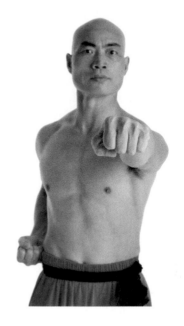

Zou! Strike with your right fist, snapping your arm up and out like you're throwing a punch straight from your shoulder. As your arm shoots out, rotate it so that when you strike, the palm of your fist is facing the ground and the back of your hand is facing the sky. Do it in one smooth, twisting extension. The twist gives the punch extra power. Think of the last time you tried to drive a nail into a hard plaster wall. It wasn't easy. You kept pounding the nail with a hammer, probably bending the nail before you made much of a dent in that hard wall. That's why a carpenter uses a screw and a power drill. *Tzzt*—in a blink, that screw digs firmly into the wall, and you're ready to hang a painting from it. It's the same principle behind this twisting punch. The twisting action gives it extra power.

Now strike the same way with the left fist, and at exactly the same moment, slide your right fist back and chamber it at your waist. As your left arm is twisting out, your right arm is twisting back. In Chinese they say, *"Gun chu, gun ru"*(滚出滚入)—"Twist out, twist in." The two arms should be moving simultaneously and in total harmony, like two screws pistoning in and out, in and out.

Do it slowly until your body gets the logic of it; then speed it up. As with the palm strikes, you'll actually find that as you begin to do it faster, you'll also be doing it more fluidly and naturally. And the faster you do it, the more powerful the punch. Snap your arms out and back with the speed of rubber bands. Right. Left. Right. Left. Remember to twist the punch like a power drill rotating a screw—*tzzt!* Punch! Retract! Punch! Retract! Punch! Retract!

Awesome! Keep practicing these two strikes, palms and fists, until they're instinctive and you can do them with real speed and power. They're integral to much of what you're going to be learning in the coming sessions.

Meditation

My body is a gift from my parents and from Buddha. I was given it to use. I will not waste this precious gift.

Our bodies are gifts from our parents and from Buddha, and we were given them to use. If you don't use your body, it becomes like an abandoned car. You can almost feel the rust forming in your joints. Then, when you need it—when you have to run to catch a bus—it won't start. That's why it's important to maintain your mental and physical condition.

As we all know, obesity has reached epidemic proportions in the United States, and it's spreading throughout the world as more and more cultures imitate Western lifestyles and diets. Sifu teaches that 21st-century technology is a fantastic gift. We don't have to walk everywhere. We can fly from the United States to China overnight. With our cellular phones, we can call anyone, anytime, from anywhere.

But at the same time, all this technology can make us lazy and overweight. As we gain weight and avoid physical exercise, our bodies fall apart. The extra pounds strain our backs, knees, ankles, and joints. We sit at computers all day, putting stress on our necks and shoulders. Day by day, the body falls apart a little more.

Without balance, a blessing can become a burden. You truly can have too much of a good thing. Let's say a person sees that a friend is having trouble walking, so she gives her a pair of new, comfortable walking shoes. That is a blessing. But suppose she gives her 10 pairs of shoes? Now she has to carry those extra 9 pairs, which makes walking a little more difficult. What if she gives her 100 pairs? How far can she walk now? The blessing has become a burden.

It's a blessing to live in a world where we're surrounded by all this technology and we have an abundance of food to eat. But if we eat too much, if we let the technology make us lazy, these blessings can very literally turn into a burden—the burden of extra weight. That extra 100 pounds you carry around every day is like those 100 pairs of shoes.

Life is so beautiful. It may seem like a long time, but it's very short. When you are a child, you have no responsibilities. Adults take care of you, give you clothes and food, keep you safe and happy. Then you leave your parents' home and go out into the world on your own. You study, you begin a career, you get married, you have kids. You may also begin to think too much, worry too much, confuse yourself, and forget to enjoy all these beautiful things that have come into your life.

Life is short. From the day you leave your parents' house to the day you die might be 40, 50, 80 years. That may seem like a long time. But subtract all the time you spend asleep during those years. All the hours you spend eating. All the days you are sick. All the holidays you spend doing nothing. All the days you wake up with no chi and don't feel like doing anything. When you take out all those days and nights, how many hours do you really have left to seriously, honestly, 100 percent express the beauty of your life?

Get up! Life is for living. Life is action. Life is exercise. We express ourselves through our actions. Our bodies are a gift from our parents and from Buddha. Don't waste the gift! Use it. Free your body and your mind. Enjoy your beautiful life every day, every hour, every second.

"AMITUOFO! AMITUOFO! AMITUOFO!"

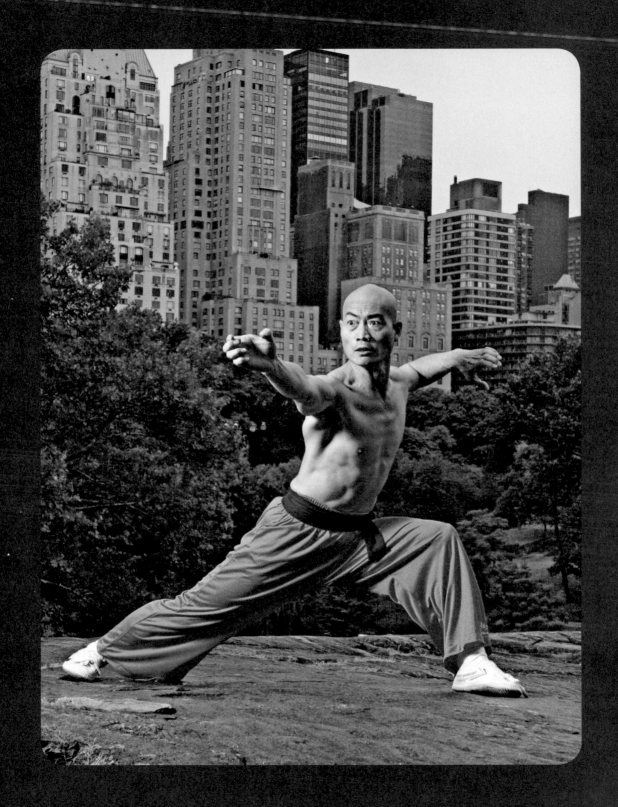

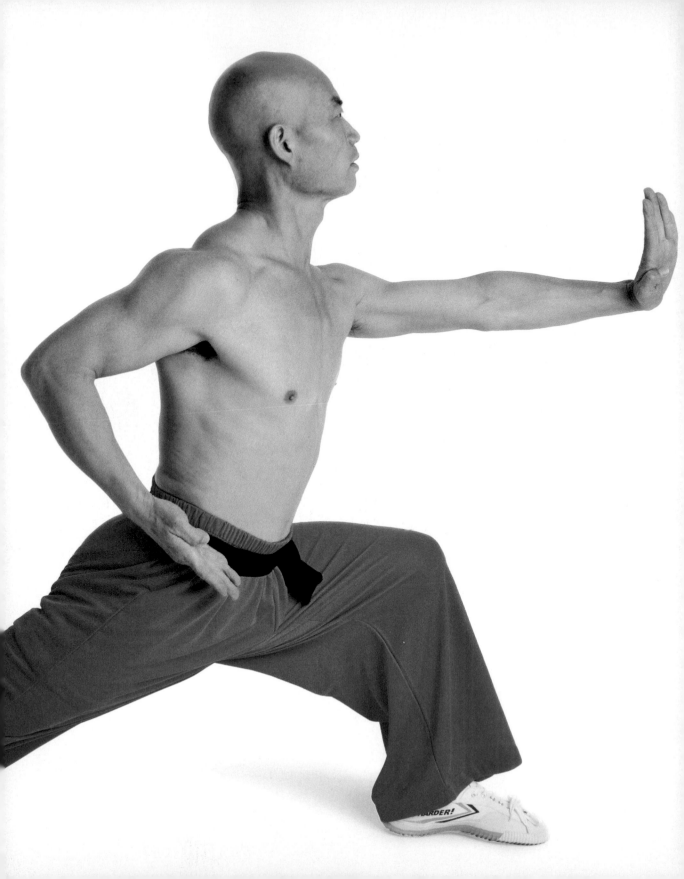

Bow Stance

"AMITUOFO!"
"AMITUOFO!"
"AMITUOFO!"

Begin with your daily routine, practicing everything you've learned.

Today things really get fun. Today you begin to understand why you've been stretching so hard, practicing your moves and your strikes so diligently every day. Because today you begin to integrate them into your first really cool set of kung fu moves, the bow stance, or Gong Bu. (*Bu* means "step.") During the rest of the Shaolin Workout, you'll learn the basic stances that are the foundation for all other kung fu movements. The kung fu student who doesn't learn these stances might as well train Iceland-style: See the polar bears, and run away!

Gong Bu is an orchestration of several movements you've already been practicing as separate elements. Take your time. Keep at it. Train harder. You'll get it. And you're going to love the feeling of accomplishment when you do.

BOW STANCE
(Gong Bu)

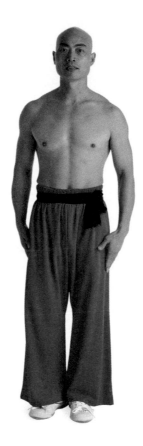

You're going to learn Gong Bu (pronounced *gung boo*) in two versions: a "traveling" version, in which you march across the room, and a stationary version, which you can do standing in one place, literally anywhere—in your bedroom, in a hotel room, at the office, in the kitchen while you're waiting for the teapot to whistle.

TRAVELING VERSION

Gong Bu coordinates several parts of your body in several movements. Think of it is as a combination of the hamstring/Gong Bu stretch you previously learned but with palm strikes. Let's break it down into separate steps.

Begin by standing straight and relaxed, with your feet close together and your hands at your sides.

Yu bei! In one quick motion, slide your hands up your legs to your waist, and chamber your fists. As you're doing that, snap your head to the left 90 degrees so that your chin is in line with your shoulder—just like you do when you're doing the eye focus exercises. See the dolphins?

Zou! Turn your whole body 90 degrees to the left, pivoting your feet without lifting or spreading them. As you turn, bring your right arm up and out at chest height. Don't extend it fully this time—bend your elbow so that your arm is curling out in front of your chest. Open that fist so that your fingers are pointing to the left, in the same gesture you learned yesterday when doing the palm strikes. And while you're opening that fist, also open your left fist so that your left hand is open

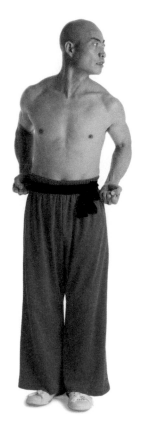

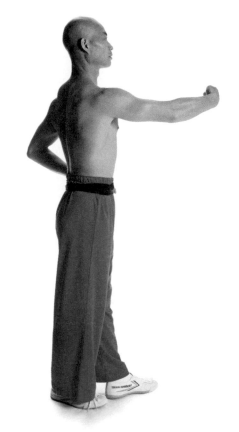

at the waist, palm up, fingers straight, thumb tucked in—five fingers together as one, as though your left hand were a knife blade you're holding at your waist, getting ready to strike. When you've completed the 90-degree turn, your whole body should be facing the dolphins. Keep your shoulders and upper body straight, your back fully extended.

Got it? Just try doing that turn slowly a few times until your body understands. Don't take a step or move your feet except to pivot them in the same spot.

Now keep adding elements. When you've completed the turn, lift your left leg in front of you, bending the knee, until your thigh is at least waist high and parallel to the

ground (higher if you can do it comfortably). Angle your raised leg to the right; this way, your left leg is defending your groin and lower body while your right arm is defending your upper body. Keep your right leg fully extended with the knee locked.

(Some students start out thinking that bending that knee will improve their balance. The opposite is in fact true—for best balance, keep that leg fully extended. Think of a skyscraper climbing 100 stories or more into the sky. Its straight walls and girders give it the strength to stand that tall. If the walls were bent or crooked, it would topple. Sifu says this is true of your whole life— the more fully you extend your life, the more you're able to find balance.)

(continued)

BOW STANCE (cont.)

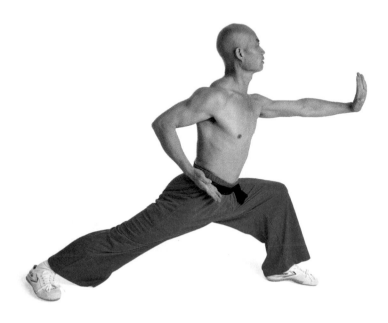

Now to complete the movement. Step down into the Gong Bu strike, bringing your left foot down with the toes pointing forward. Your thigh should be parallel to the ground, or lower if you can. At exactly the same time, strike with your left palm. Your left palm should complete the strike as your left foot lands. Strike quickly, with chi—pow! Sifu says that when you strike, move the mountain! As you strike with the left hand, slide your right palm back to your waist, the blade of your fingers pointing forward, palm toward the sky.

Just as in the Gong Bu stretches you've been practicing, you should fully extend your body when you strike, with your chest forward, your back straight, your head and chin up. Don't lean over your left leg—extend your upper body toward the sky. Your right leg should be extended

straight behind you, knee locked, right foot firmly planted on the ground and pointed as close to parallel with your other foot as you comfortably can. Remember also to close your groin when you strike.

Practice this move until your body understands it. Pivot, raise your left leg and left arm, step down into the Gong Bu strike, and strike with left palm while your left foot hits the ground. Do it again. And again. Got the idea? Good!

So we continue. Let's "travel." To do that, we alternate left strike/left leg, right strike/right leg.

Do the entire move, from the beginning, striking to the left. Now, from that position, turn your left hand so that the fingers are pointed 90 degrees to your right. At the

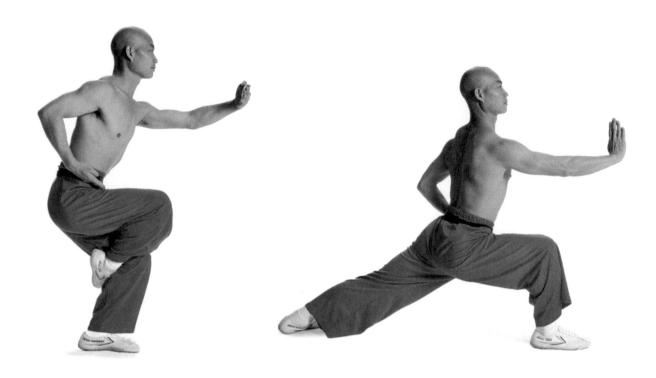

same time, lift your *right* leg and tuck your right foot behind the left knee, keeping the left knee bent. Do this without lifting your body to standing height—stay down at striking height.

Go down into a Gong Bu strike with your right foot, striking with your right palm as you do. While you strike with the right palm, the left one slides to your left waist.

Do you see why this is called the "traveling" version of Gong Bu? From where you started, you've taken two steps toward the dolphins, executing a palm strike with each step, first left hand/leg and then right hand/leg. You could keep marching like this all the way to Miami, pushing that mountain into the ocean! Strike left, strike right, strike left.

Yes, Gong Bu is definitely the most complex series of moves you've learned yet. It is also among the few most important stances in all martial arts. Anyone who practices the martial arts must understand Gong Bu. Do you see how all you're doing is combining elements you've already been practicing separately? This is what you have been practicing them for; now you're combining them in beautiful harmony and coordination. Don't worry if you mess up at first, confuse the movements, lose your balance. You will master them if you want to. Practice really does make perfect.

As you're getting the sequence of moves down, keep perfecting your form. Fully extend your arms, your legs, your upper body. Keep your shoulders straight, your chest and head high. Keep your groin closed. Feel the chi flowing all the way into the edge of your palm when you strike. Move the mountain!

(continued)

BOW STANCE (cont.)

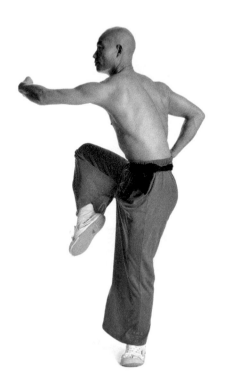
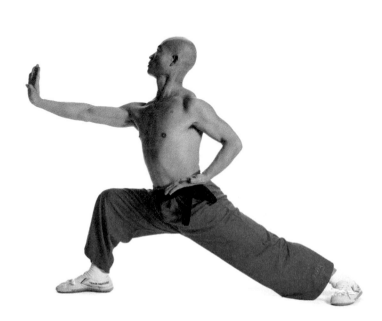

STATIONARY VERSION

If you're doing the Shaolin Workout in your bedroom, hotel room, or office, you're going to palm-strike a wall long before you reach the dolphins. There were many times over the centuries when the Shaolin monks were outlawed and had to practice their moves in small places, too, in secret, at the dead of night. That's why they say, *"Quan da wo hu zhi di"* (拳打臥虎之地)—"You can practice kung fu in the space a tiger lies down in." So there's a standing-in-one-place version of Gong Bu.

First, execute a Gong Bu strike to your left. Now, instead of continuing to march in that direction,

you're going to turn around and strike in the opposite direction. Turn your body to the right, pivoting your left foot and coming around 180 degrees. At the same time, curl your left arm around in front of your chest as you lift your right leg, with your knee bent and groin closed.

Now strike, bringing your right foot down as you strike with your right hand. Fully extend your entire body, and strike with snap and chi.

Now you can turn back again toward the dolphins. Pivot your right foot, turning your body 180 degrees

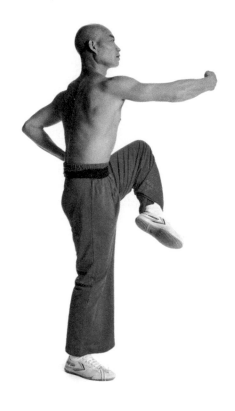

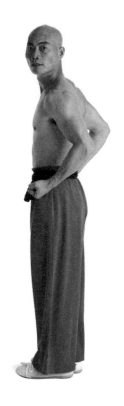

to the left while you curl your right arm around in front of your chest. Lift your left leg at the same time. Strike with your left palm as you plant your left foot.

See? You just struck in both directions, to the left and to the right, without moving away from your starting position. Practice until it's natural and you don't have to think about it.

Beautiful! You look like a real kung fu warrior! Uma Thurman would be jealous.

Note: Don't feel frustrated if you find your feet getting tangled at first or you forget which hand strikes with which foot. Your body will learn with practice and repetition. Don't think about it too hard, or your feet may trip over your brain! If you worry too much about learning Gong Bu, you won't get to sleep tonight, and tomorrow you'll have no chi for training harder.

Keep at it. Soon you'll be executing Gong Bu as naturally as you walk. With dedicated training, it will become that instinctive.

Meditation

Everyone has Buddha inside him or her.

There are almost 7 billion people living today in the world. Chan Buddhism teaches that this means there are 7 billion Buddhas on earth right now. That's because Buddhists believe that Buddha lives in each and every one of us and that all things in the universe can become Buddha.

You don't need to be a Buddhist to see the beauty and truth of this concept. Sifu believes that there are as many paths to enlightenment as there are living beings. Each of us must create his or her own path. It doesn't matter which spiritual leader you follow. Buddha, Moses, Jesus, Muhammad, and the other great spiritual leaders all teach us the same simple truths: to do good, and not to do bad; to help yourself, help others, and help the world; to spread peace, love, respect, and understanding.

Chan Buddhists believe you have Buddha in your heart, just like people in the West say you have God in your heart. That's why you should love and respect each and every person, just as you love and respect yourself. Buddha, or God, created this beautiful universe and your wonderful life. You must truly understand and appreciate that gift.

"AMITUOFO! AMITUOFO! AMITUOFO!"

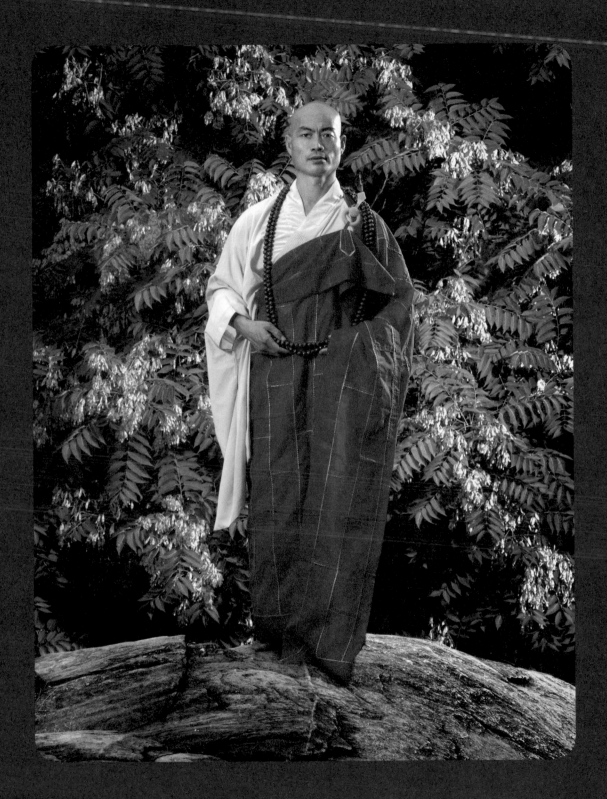

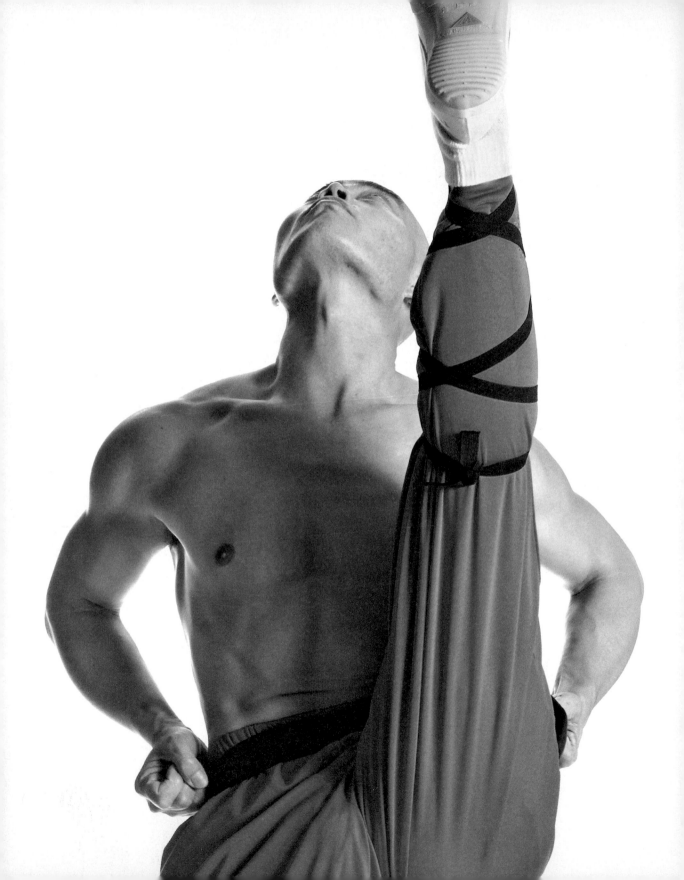

Front Slap Kick

"AMITUOFO!"

"AMITUOFO!"

"AMITUOFO!"

Begin with your usual routine, running through all your exercises and moves, from the wrist stretch to Gong Bu.

FRONT SLAP KICK
(Caijiao)

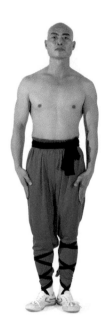 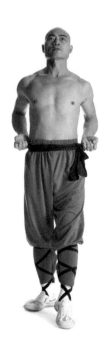 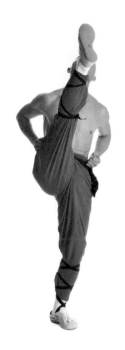

Yesterday you learned your first stance. Today learn your first kick. It incorporates both your legs and your arms, so let's break it down.

Just learn the legs first. You can start with either foot, but for this example start with a right-leg kick.

Stand straight and relaxed, feet together.

Yu bei! Quickly chamber your fists at your waist, and at the same time take a small step forward with your left leg, foot fully extended, onto your toes. Keep both knees locked and your body fully extended from your toes to the top of your head. If you have hair, your hair should be extended, too!

Now you're going to kick with your right leg.

Zou! In one smooth move, keeping both legs straight and both knees locked, kick your right leg straight up in front of you as you plant your left foot firmly on the ground. Your right foot should be fully extended so that your toes are in a straight line with your leg. Kick up as high and as quickly as you can *without* bending your knee or leaning your body forward. When the kick reaches its highest point, lower your leg at the same speed as you kicked up. Your foot should land on the toes. At the same time, extend your body even higher than before—reach for enlightenment with the top of your head!

Try that right-leg kick a few times. It's critical not to bend your knee. Your leg should scissor straight up from the hip, up as high as you can kick, toes pointed, and then down until your toes touch the ground. When those toes touch the ground, all your weight should be

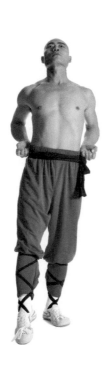
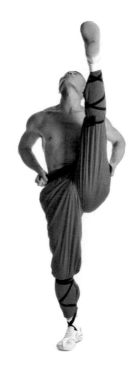
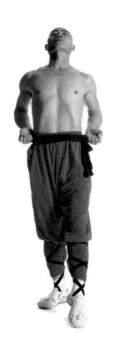

on your other leg. Touch your toes lightly to the ground. As you master Caijiao (pronounced *sy-jow*) and the other kicks in the Shaolin Workout, try to express an explosion of chi at the top of every kick, like the crack of a whip—pow! Sifu says that when you kick, it should be like lightning, and when your toes touch down, it should be as light as a feather.

Now learn to kick with both legs—right, left, right, left—kick-marching across the ground.

Yu bei! Assume the ready position, left foot forward on its toes.

Zou! Kick with the right leg. This time, don't stop when the toes of your right foot touch the ground. Go directly into a left-leg kick. Your right toes touch the ground. Your right heel comes down to the ground as your left

foot kicks up off the ground. Kick as high and fast with your left leg as you can, knee locked, toes pointing straight out in line with the leg. Crack the whip at the top of the kick—pow! Then bring that foot down lightly on its toes.

Keep going—marching forward, kicking with every step. Your left toes touch the ground, left heel comes down as you kick up with the right leg. Right leg comes down; left leg kicks up. Don't pause between kicks. Kick-march toward the dolphins. Kick left! Kick right! Kick left! Kick right! Don't stop! Don't stop! Don't lean forward. Back straight! Head up! Chest forward! Shoulders square! How high can you kick without bending your knees? Kick like you're trying to kick the leaves off the tops of the trees.

Fabulous.

(continued)

FRONT SLAP KICK (cont.)

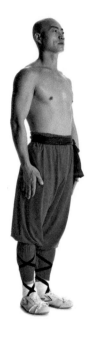 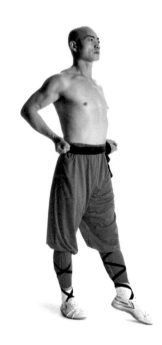 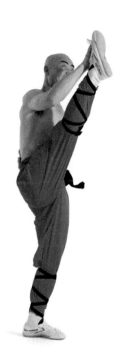

Now add the final element—your arms.

Yu bei! Assume the ready position: left leg forward, toes to ground, knee locked, fists chambered at waist.

Zou! Kick straight up with your right leg. At the same time, as quickly as you execute a strike, extend your right arm and slap your foot at the highest point of the kick. Then, with the same speed, chamber that fist at your

waist as you lower that leg to the toes. Really snap that arm out and back like a rubber band—pow! Don't forget to fully extend your body when your foot lands.

Understand? Practice it a few times.

Now travel. Execute a slap kick with the right foot. As soon as the right toes touch the ground, execute a left kick, snapping your left hand out and back to slap

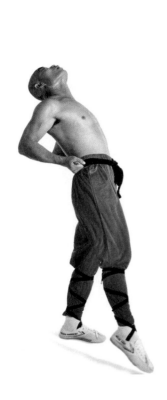 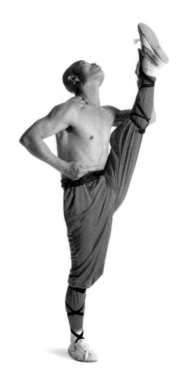 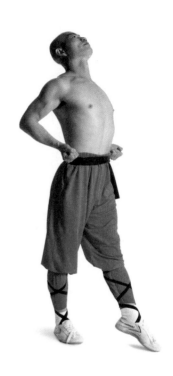

that foot at the peak of the kick. As the left toes land, go into a right slap kick. And so on, marching toward the dolphins.

If you don't have space to march around in, you can practice these kicks in one spot. Kick right, kick left, kick right, without traveling.

Don't feel bad if at first your leg can't get up high enough to reach your hand. You'll get there with practice. So don't cheat by leaning forward, by bending your knees, or by lifting your heel off the ground. Don't worry about going slow. Just keep moving forward every day, challenging yourself, encouraging yourself, mastering yourself.

Day by day, you will kick higher, faster, and stronger, no question.

Meditation

If I run away from my problems, they will only follow me and defeat me.

If you run away from a problem or a challenge, it's not going to disappear. It will follow you and defeat you.

Today, stand and face your problems and challenges, whatever they are. For example, let's say you're having a problem in your marriage or relationship. Sometimes people don't face a problem and don't communicate with each other about it. They both pretend to ignore it and hope it just goes away. But that problem, whatever it is, won't simply disappear. If the two of you don't face it and fix it together, it will live with you and intrude on your life together. Remind yourselves of the first day you met. You looked so handsome and beautiful to each other. You cherished and loved each other so much. You respected each other so deeply. Where are those two people now?

Imagine you're a fighter in a ring. The other fighter wants nothing more than to beat you up. You must have the confidence to face him and take the blows so that you can fight back. If you turn away and don't face him, you'll never see him coming, and he'll be free to punch you, kick you, slap you, bite your ear—whatever he wants! That fighter is a problem you're not facing.

Think of your Shaolin Workout training. If you can't face a bit of pain or a sore muscle, that becomes a problem that will never go away, and you'll never make progress and transform your life. Don't turn away from it. Don't think about it—just do it!

"AMITUOFO! AMITUOFO! AMITUOFO!"

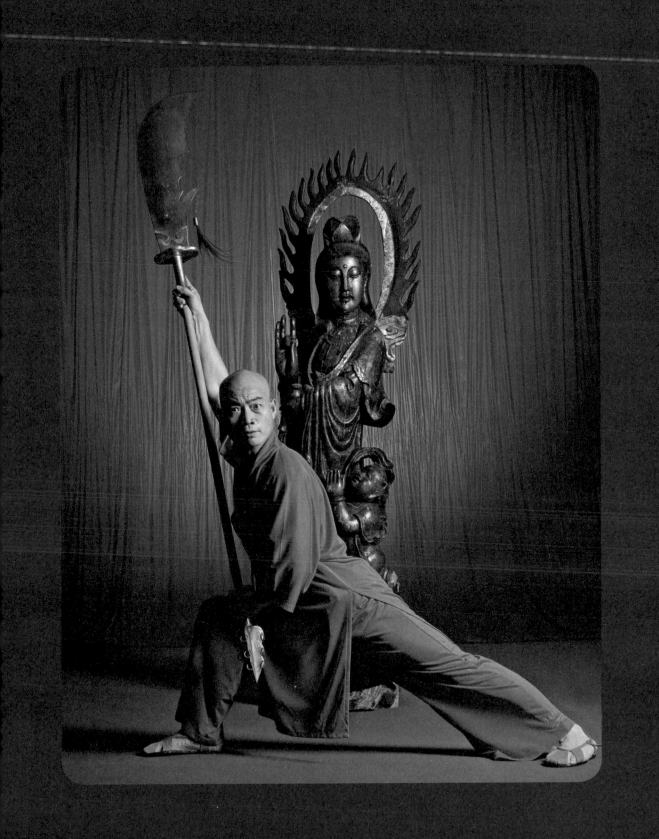

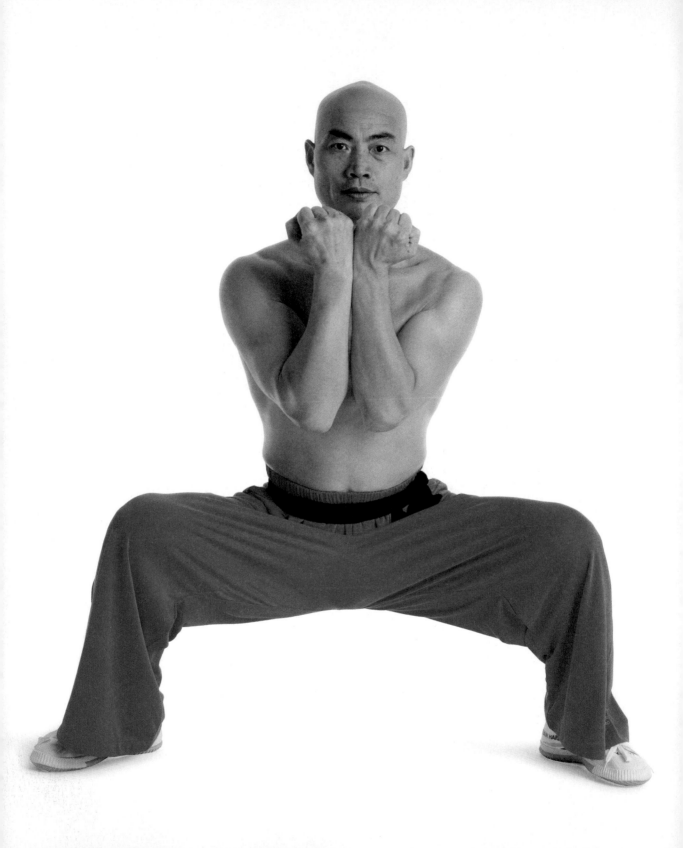

Horse Stance

"AMITUOFO!"
"AMITUOFO!"
"AMITUOFO!"

Go through your entire routine. More chi! Train harder!

HORSE STANCE
(Ma Bu)

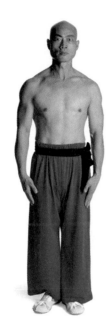
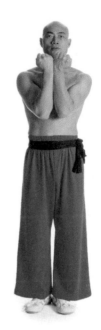

Today, learn another stance: Ma Bu (pronounced *mah boo*), the horse stance. You will learn three versions of Ma Bu: a traveling version, a one-step version, and a stationary version.

TRAVELING VERSION
Ma Bu incorporates steps, fist punches, and head movements. Learn the traveling version first, in stages, beginning with the arms.

Stand straight and relaxed, feet close together, hands at your sides.

In one smooth movement, squeeze your shoulders and tuck your arms in front of you so that your elbows are together in front of your stomach, your forearms are together in a straight line perpendicular to your chest,

and your fists are together, the backs of your hands facing out, the edges of your palms pressed together. Tuck your chin. It's like a boxer blocking punches. The tops of your fists should be about at chin height. Don't raise them so high that you can't see past your knuckles. Look straight out in front of you as far as you can. Look all the way to your beautiful future.

Now you will strike—a double strike, using both fists at the same time. In one swift move, punch out to the left and right *simultaneously*, snapping your arms out to your sides at shoulder height.

Think of it as two side fist punches executed simultaneously; instead of punching straight in front of you, one fist at a time, you're punching straight out to your sides, both fists at the same time. Your arms should fully

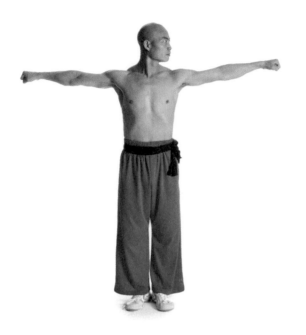
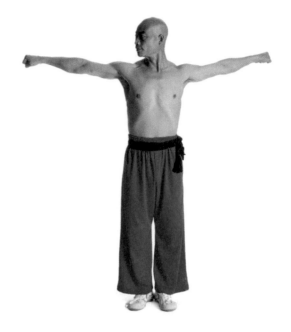

extend in a single straight line out through the shoulders from fist to fist. Your elbows should be locked. Fully extend your upper body and open your chest wide when you strike. Pow!

Your head and eyes are involved as well. You're punching your fists out in both directions simultaneously—but who are you punching? You need to look, in both directions, very quickly. When you start to strike, you start to move your head so that your arms and your head finish at exactly the same instant. As you punch your fists out, snap your head to the left and then to your right in one quick movement: Look left—boom—right!

Your head should be completing the move just as your fists complete the punch. At the end of this double punch, your fists will be fully extended to either side at

shoulder height, and your head will be turned 90 degrees to the right so that your chin is over your right shoulder.

Got that? Now try it again, only alternating the direction of your head snaps. Bring your arms back together in front of you, elbows and forearms together, fists at your chin. Now strike! As your fists punch out, look quickly to your right, then left. Right—boom—left! At the end of the strike, your head should be turned 90 degrees to the left this time, chin over left shoulder.

Practice the strike, alternating the left and right head turns. Let's do it 10 times. *Yi*—right. *Er*—left. *San*—right. *Si*—left. . . .

Fantastic.

(continued)

HORSE STANCE (cont.)

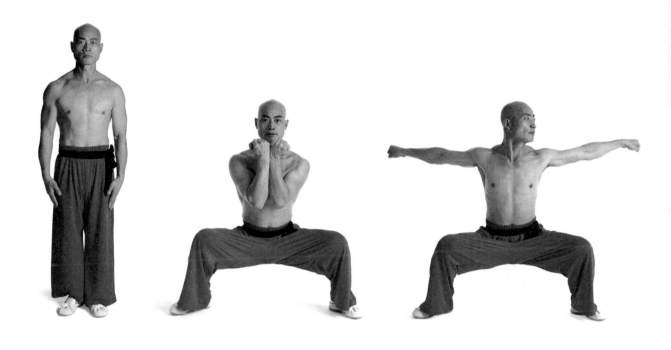

Add the legs. Stand straight and relaxed, with your feet close together and your hands at your sides.

Now you're going to lower yourself into a squat. Keeping your left foot firm and flat, take a comfortable step to the right with your right foot. Keep your body facing forward. Don't turn your body, and don't move your left foot at all. Just take a step to the right with your right foot.

At the same time that you start to step to the right, begin to lift your arms in front of you the way you've just been practicing, with your elbows and forearms together and your fists at your chin. Your arms and your legs should complete their moves at exactly the same instant.

As your right foot steps down flat to the ground, bend both of your knees and come down in a squat. Squat so

that your thighs are parallel to the ground. Your legs and hips should be wide-open so that your knees are aiming in opposite directions, one knee pointing to the dolphins, the other pointing to the polar bears. Your toes should be pointing forward. As you complete the squat, bring your arms together in front of you.

Your upper body will be suspended directly in the middle, equidistant from your knees. Keep your back straight and fully extended—don't lean forward. Hold your head high and straight. Think of your head as a bell suspended by a chain straight up to the sky. Also, don't stick your buttocks out behind you. This will cause your upper body to lean forward. Lift your butt and tuck it in tight. You should be one straight, perpendicular line from the back of your head down your spine and to your buttocks. Another way to think of this is that your three chi centers—your Dentien in Chinese (丹田)—should be perfectly in line. Your upper

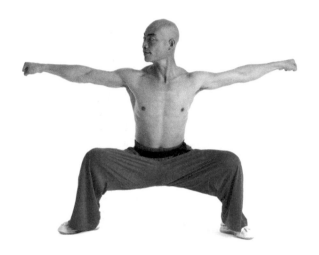

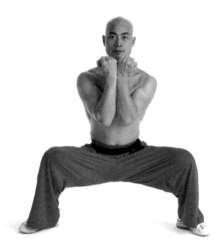

Dentien is the spot in the center of your forehead, between your eyebrows. Your middle Dentien is the spot in the center of your chest. And straight down from that, exactly 1.3 inches below your navel, is your third Dentien. They should form a straight line perpendicular to the ground.

Practice taking that step to the right and bringing your arms together in front of you until you've got it. Remember to keep your upper body fully extended.

Stand, relax, and practice stepping to the left with the left foot. It's the same actions, just to the left.

Got it? Beautiful.

Now add the strikes. Let's begin by stepping to the right. Stand and relax, with your hands at your sides. Take a step to the right with your right foot and go

down into the squat. At the same time, bring your arms together in front of you, with your fists at your chin. Remember to keep your upper body fully extended and to tuck in your butt. Look far out over your knuckles and see your future.

Strike with both fists simultaneously, and at the same time snap your head left, then right. Bam!

Practice this right step and strike until you've got it. Alternate the direction of your head snaps as you repeat the step—first left-right, then right-left, then left-right again.

Practice the exact same moves, only stepping to the left with your left foot.

Fabulous! You look like a fierce warrior riding into battle, clocking your attackers on both sides as your horse charges through them.

(continued)

HORSE STANCE (cont.)

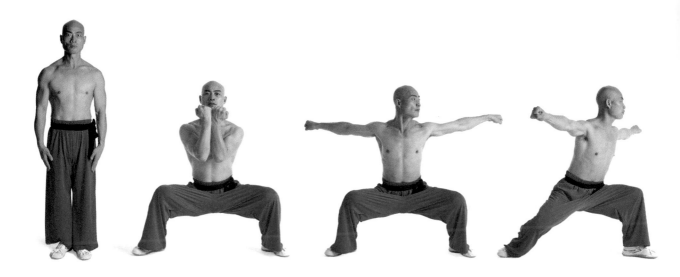

Now learn how to travel. You can begin in either direction, but for this example let's start with a right step. Stand straight and relaxed, hands at your sides. Take your step to the right and go into your squat, at the same time as you bring your arms together in front of you. Look far out over your knuckles; then strike—pow!—snapping your head left, then right.

Now you travel. Pivot on your *left* foot and simultaneously lift your *right* foot and tuck it behind your left knee as you turn your whole body around in a *forward* (counterclockwise) arc. Come around 180 degrees, until you're facing the opposite direction from where you just started the pivot. Bring your right foot down flat, toes pointing forward. Don't lift your body as you execute this pivoting turn—stay down in the squat. Also, as you're turning, don't drop your arms—keep them up and extended at shoulder height in the strike position.

Then, as your right foot steps down to the ground, swiftly fold your arms together in front of you, elbows together, fists at chin height. Look far ahead for an instant. Now strike, snapping your head right, then left.

Keep traveling in the same direction. Pivot on your *right* foot this time, tucking your left foot behind your right knee, and turn your body 180 degrees in a forward (now clockwise) arc. Remember not to rise out of the squat, and to keep your arms extended in the strike position when you are turning. As you step down with your left foot, bring your arms together in front of you. Look straight ahead. Now strike, snapping your head left, then right.

Understand? Practice this traveling version of Ma Bu until your body gets it. Remember to keep your upper body fully extended and your three Dentiens aligned. And never lift out of the squat as you travel.

Magnificent!

(continued)

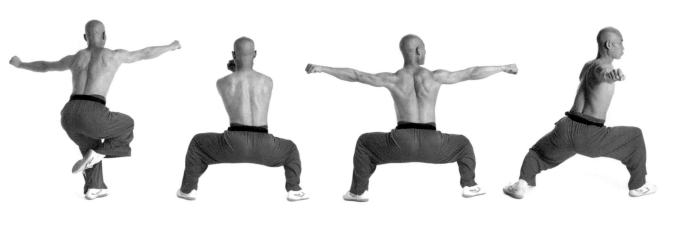

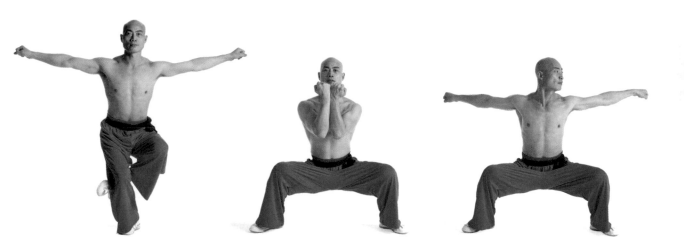

HORSE STANCE (cont.)

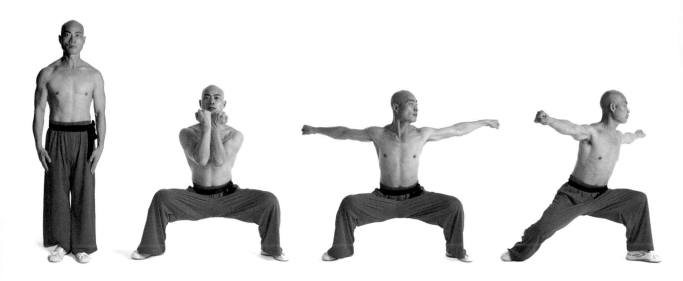

ONE-STEP VERSION

Just as with Gong Bu, you could keep squat-marching Ma Bu strikes all the way to the dolphins. But you're going to run into a wall or a fence before you reach them. So there are versions of Ma Bu you can do in smaller spaces.

First, the one-step version.

Go down into the squat, and strike. Pivot on one foot—let's make it the left for this example. Turn your body in a forward (counterclockwise) arc 180 degrees, and strike.

Now pivot on the *same* foot, the left one, and turn your body around another 180 degrees in a forward (counterclockwise) arc. When you complete the turn, strike. Remember to alternate the head snaps, left-right, right-left.

See? You just executed two Ma Bu strikes, facing in opposite directions without moving from one spot. Your pivot foot never leaves the ground and is always in the same spot.

Practice this version 10 times. *Yi*—pivot-strike. *Er*—pivot-strike. *San*—pivot-strike. *Si*—pivot-strike.

(continued)

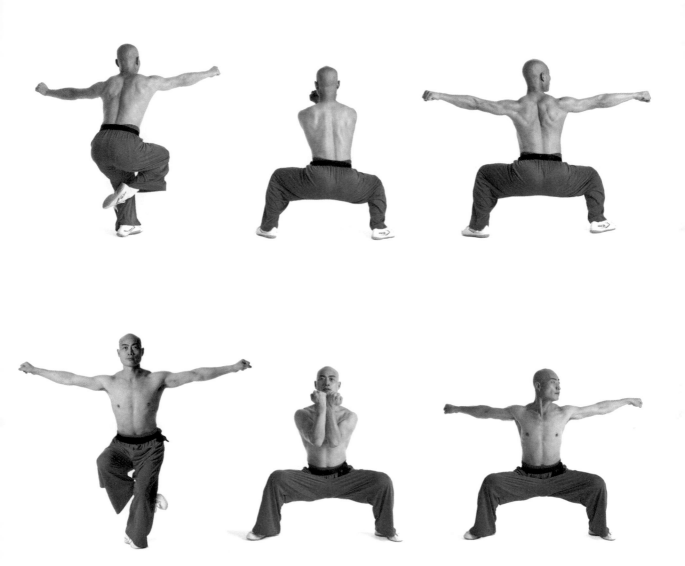

HORSE STANCE (cont.)

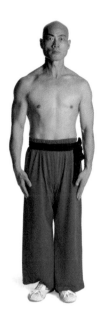 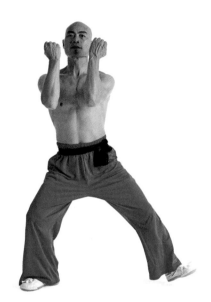 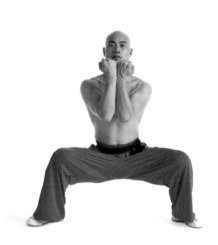

STATIONARY VERSION

You can practice Ma Bu without moving your feet at all—in your bedroom, a hotel room, the office, a bus stop or subway platform, or on top of the conference room table during a long conference call! Go into the squat and execute the fist punches, snapping your head—pow! Maintain the squat. Don't move your body or feet at all. Just tuck your arms back in to the chest position, fists at chin. Look far ahead. Punch again. And repeat. You can keep repeating these punches for as long as you can hold the squat. Alternate the direction of your head snaps each time. Look right-left, then left-right, then right-left. . . . Practice this 10 times.

You look striking! Keep practicing these variations of Ma Bu until the end of your session today. When you're done, you'll feel new strength in your thighs, buttocks, shoulders, and arms. Feels wonderful, doesn't it? It looks wonderful, too.

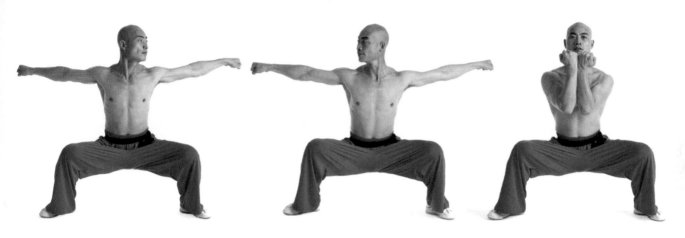

Meditation

My life is a work of art, and I am the artist.

Our bodies are beautiful, like music or works of art. Our bodies have rhythm and melodies, like music. They have beauty and form, like art. Living is an art form. You create your life the way an artist expresses herself through a sculpture or a song. When you exercise your body and your mind, building physical and mental strength and discipline, you're sculpting yourself into a beautiful work of art. That's why they call it martial *arts.* You're polishing your body, polishing your mind, and polishing your life.

What kind of artwork do you want to be? Create it!

"AMITUOFO! AMITUOFO! AMITUOFO!"

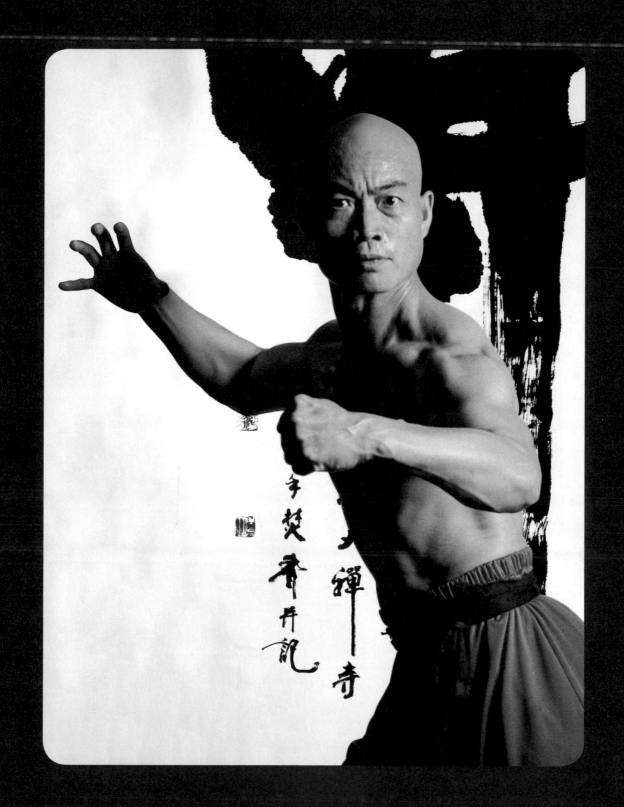

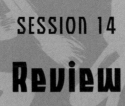

SESSION 14

Review

"AMITUOFO!"
"AMITUOFO!"
"AMITUOFO!"

Today go through everything you've been learning and practicing so far. Look at how much you've learned! Only 2 weeks ago, you might have known nothing about kung fu. Today you're practicing these beautiful, complex strikes, stances, and kicks. How cool is that? Go ahead and feel proud of what you've accomplished.

Today is the midway point in your Shaolin Workout training. In the coming sessions, you will teach yourself some amazing moves that just a couple of weeks ago you never would have believed you could do. Stay determined. Stay disciplined. Stay relaxed and focused. Keep training. Go through your entire routine every day. Feel how great it is to keep improving at it, perfecting your forms, stretching a little farther every day, kicking a little higher, punching a little faster. More chi! Train harder!

In the first half of the Shaolin Workout, you've seen yourself accomplish things you never would have believed you could. Take that sense of self-respect and apply it to your whole life. There is nothing you cannot accomplish if you want to.

"AMITUOFO!"
"AMITUOFO!"
"AMITUOFO!"

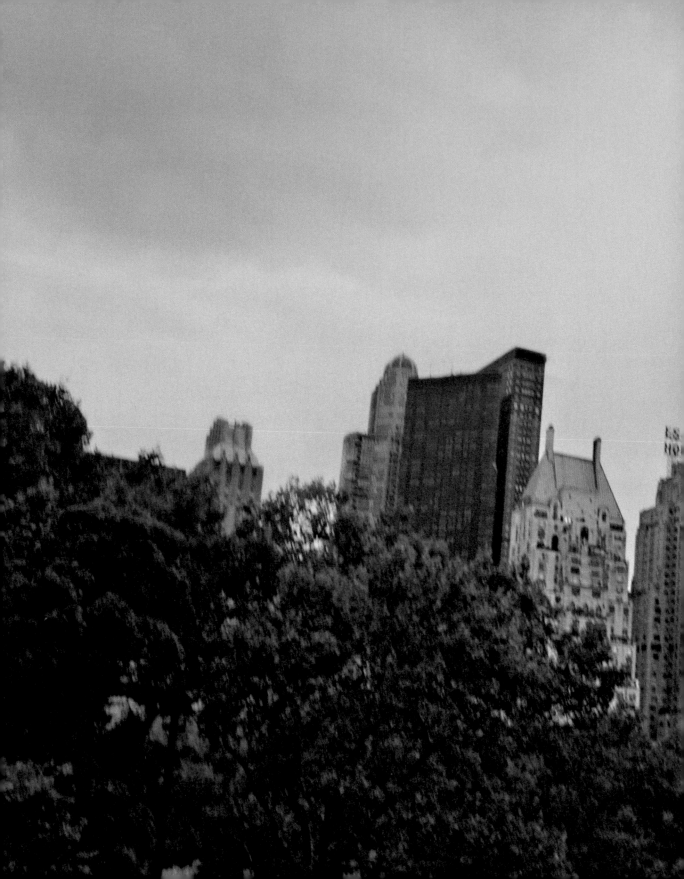

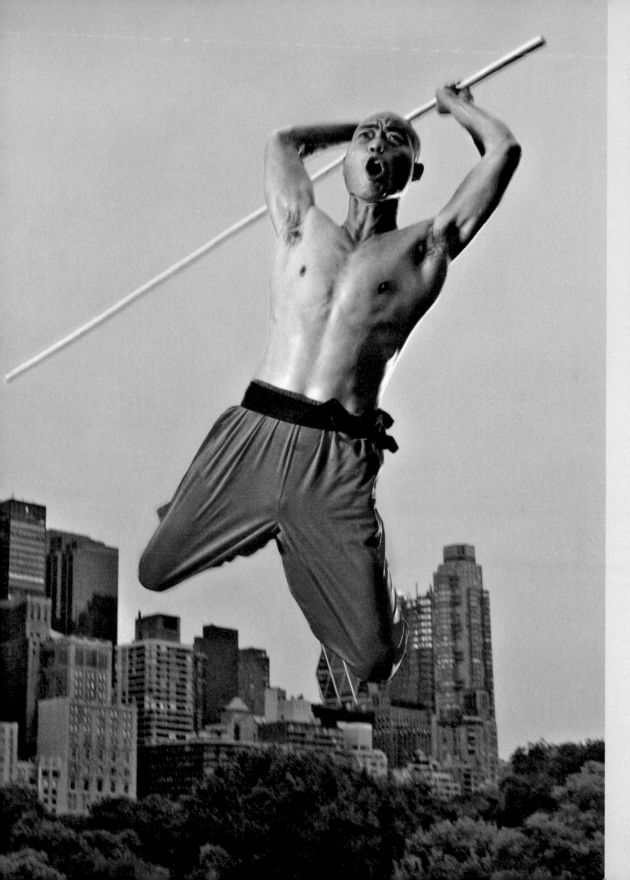

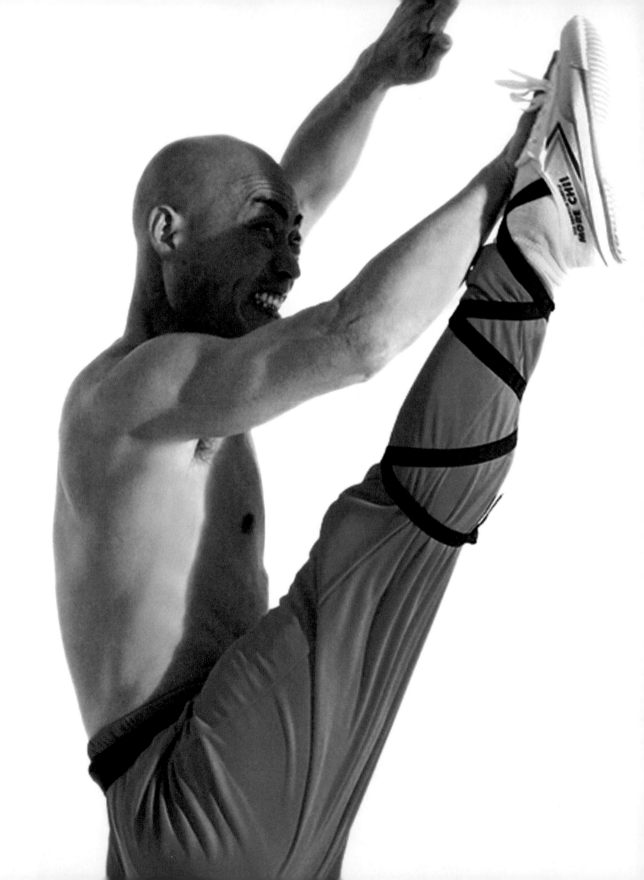

Front Slap Kick
with Arm Rotation

"AMITUOFO!"
"AMITUOFO!"
"AMITUOFO!"

Begin with all your usual training, up through Session 13. Now let's learn a new kick.

FRONT SLAP KICK WITH ARM ROTATION
(Lunbi Caijiao)

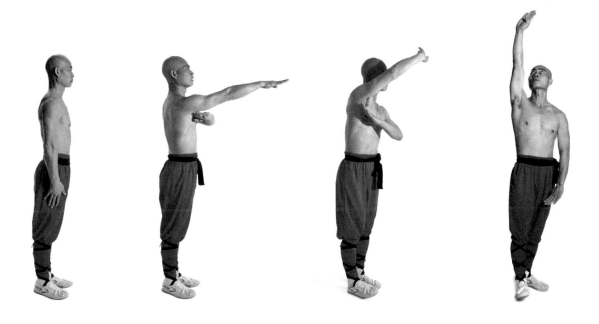

This is a variation on Caijiao, the front slap kick you learned in Session 12. Lunbi Caijiao (pronounced *lun-bee sy-jow*) adds arm movements based on the arm rotations you've been doing since way back in Session 3. Learn it in steps, beginning with the arms.

Stand straight and relaxed, feet together, your body fully extended.

Yu bei! Hold your right arm straight out in front of you at shoulder height, palm flat and facing the ground, fingers pointing straight ahead. Cross your left arm in front of your chest and place the palm of your left hand in your right armpit, palm toward the ground.

Zou! Without taking a step or opening your stance, turn your body 90 degrees to the right, pivoting on both feet. When you begin to turn, also begin to rotate your arms. Slide your left arm down the front of your body and then up until it's straight out to the left side from your shoulder.

Simultaneously, rotate your right arm up and out to the side until it is also pointing straight out to the right. Follow your right arm with your head to the right, snapping your chin over your shoulder so that you're looking straight down your right arm to your fingertips and beyond. Complete your pivot, your arm rotation, and your head snap all together at the exact same moment.

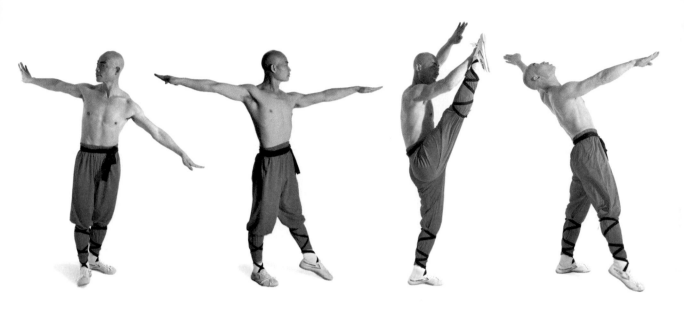

Now pivot to the left, turning back the way you were originally facing, and at the same time take a small step forward with your left foot, landing on your toes. As you pivot, keep your left arm rigid and unmoving, the fingers pointing in exactly the same spot through this whole turn. Rotate your right arm down close to your body and up toward your left arm, at the same time that you begin to kick with your right leg. Keep your knee locked, your foot and leg fully extended, the toes of your right foot pointed.

Now you slap-kick: Slap your left palm with the back of your right hand, and almost simultaneously slap your right foot with your right palm. From the slap, quickly

extend your left arm to your side, palm down, and 155 degrees from your body. Simultaneously lower your right leg to land lightly on its toes. When you slap-kick, extend your entire body up. Reach for enlightenment with the top of your head. Slap-kick with explosive, whip-cracking power—pow!—and pop your body into fullest extension. Don't cheat by leaning your body forward or lowering your left palm. You'd only be cheating yourself.

Understand? Practice it now. If it helps, learn it in stages. Repeat the pivoting turns and arm rotations first, until your body has learned them. Then add the slap kick.

(continued)

FRONT SLAP KICK WITH ARM ROTATION (cont.)

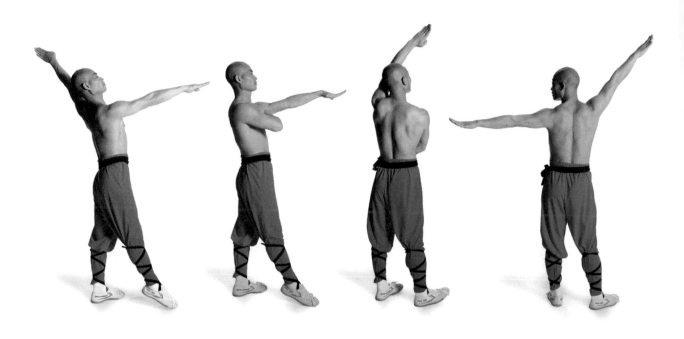

Now practice traveling, kicking only with the right leg.

Learn to travel, alternating right and left kicks. The left kick is simply the reverse of the right kick you've been practicing.

Execute a right kick. When your right toes land, leave your foot there—don't bring your feet together—and extend your *left* arm straight out in front of you at shoulder height, and place the palm of your *right* hand in your left armpit, palm toward the ground.

Pivot and turn your body 90 degrees to the *left*. When you begin to turn, also begin to rotate your arms. Slide your *right* arm down the front of your body and then up until it's straight out to the right side from your shoulder. Simultaneously, rotate your *left* arm up and out to the side until it is pointing straight out to the left. Follow your left arm with your head to the left, snapping your chin over your shoulder so that you're looking straight down your left arm to your fingertips and beyond. Complete your pivot, your arm rotation, and your head snap at the exact same moment.

Pivot to the right, turning back the way you were originally facing. As you pivot, keep your right arm rigid

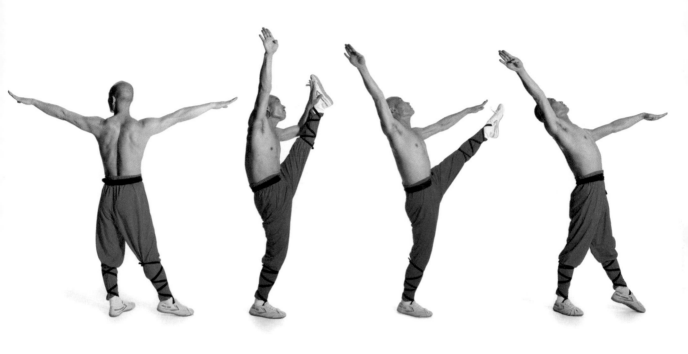

and unmoving, the fingers pointing in exactly the same spot through this whole turn. Rotate your left arm down close to your body and up toward your right arm as you begin to kick with your left leg.

Now you slap-kick: Slap your right palm with the back of your left hand, and almost simultaneously slap your left foot with your left palm. From the slap, you quickly extend your right arm to your side, palm down, 155 degrees from your body, and simultaneously lower your left leg to land lightly on its toes.

Got it? Now you can kick with your right leg again, and then the left, and then the right, slap-kicking your way to the dolphins.

Practice traveling with alternating right and left Lunbi Caijiao kicks until your body understands it. Remember at all times to keep your form sharp, your body fully extended. Add speed and power as you learn it, and try to express that explosion of chi at the moment of the slap kick. You'll feel proud of learning another beautiful kick, and you'll feel it strengthening and toning your whole body, from your toes to the top of your head.

Meditation

Paradise is inside me.

We all love to go away on vacation. To sit on some sunny beach, drink some cold "special water," watch the dolphins play in the waves, plant our toes in the sand, and have nothing to do but rest. "This is paradise!" we sigh happily.

But why do we love it so? Because it's a change from our daily routine. If all you ever did was sit on the beach every day of your whole life, with nothing to do, nothing ever changing, no mental stimulation, day in and day out for your entire life, it's guaranteed you'd go screaming mad with boredom.

Each of us has the power to create our own paradise. Paradise is not some beach on a distant island or some other plane of existence. Paradise is within you, in your heart and in your mind. Paradise is right here, wherever you are! Sifu says that the U.S.A. Shaolin Temple is Paradise Island, right in the heart of Manhattan.

You create your own life. You make it heaven or hell.

Destiny is not something that happens to you. You make your own destiny. The foolish person waits for good things to happen to him, as though he's going to wake up one morning and find the bed showered with $100 bills. If fortune and success just came to us, all the casinos in Las Vegas would be out of business. Fortune, success, happiness—they rarely just fall in your lap. You must grasp your life and sharpen it.

When you open your heart and mind to the world, the whole world opens up to you. When you polish your body and mind, you polish your life. You radiate calm, confidence, and peace. You're living in harmony and balance, wherever you are. *That's* paradise!

"AMITUOFO! AMITUOFO! AMITUOFO!"

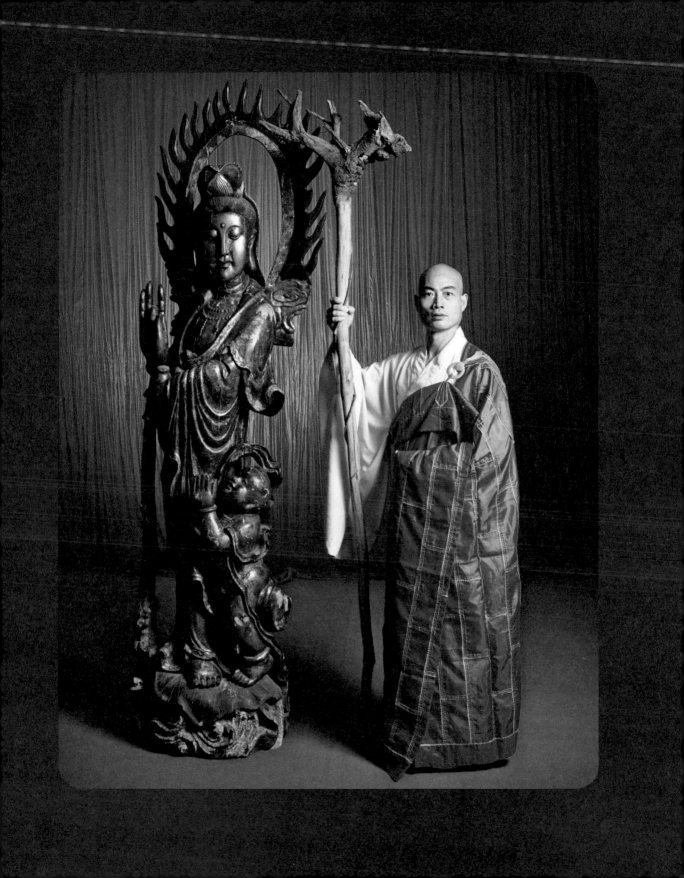

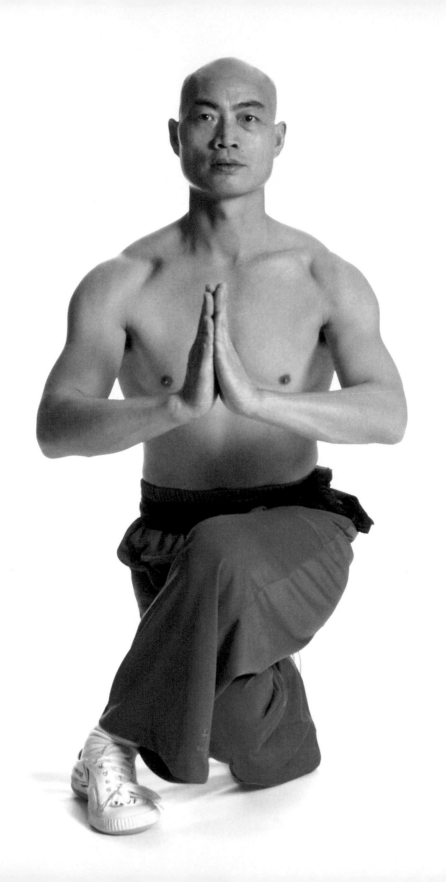

SESSION 16
Half-Crossed Seated Stance

"AMITUOFO!"

"AMITUOFO!"

"AMITUOFO!"

Execute your entire routine, from wrist rotations up through Lunbi Caijiao. Notice how you're improving every single session? Applause, applause.

HALF-CROSSED SEATED STANCE
(Xie Bu)

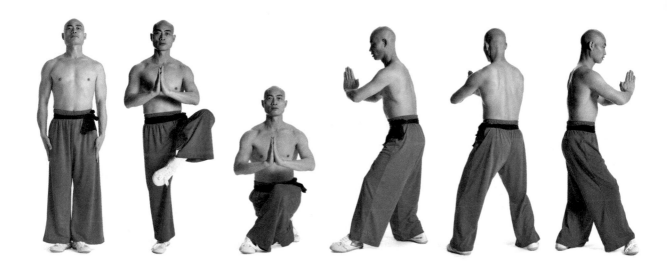

This beautiful sequence of moves, called Xie Bu (pronounced *shee-eh boo*), involves crouching and striking to one side, then turning your entire body to crouch and strike to the opposite side, and then turning back to crouch and strike from the original position. It requires coordinating your arms, legs, head, and body. Let's break it down into its separate elements, beginning with the legs and then the arms and body and head; then we'll put the pieces together.

Stand straight and relaxed, feet together. You're not going to use your arms yet, so just put your palms in front of your chest like you're praying or meditating.

Lift your left foot across your right shin, knee bent. Bend both your knees and plant your left foot in front of the right, with the toes pointing 45 degrees to the left. Crouch, with your legs crossed and your left knee over your right, as low as you can without losing your balance. But don't let your knees touch the ground.

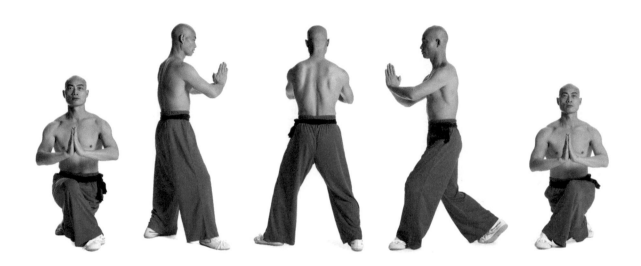

As always, keep your upper body straight and fully extended, your shoulders squared and your head up.

Got it? Practice this step until you can do it smoothly and firmly, without wobbling like you're doing Sleeping Style kung fu!

Now learn to turn and pivot. Execute the cross-legged crouch you've been practicing, with your left knee over your right. Pivot on your feet to turn your body to the right, making a 360-degree turn so that you're facing front again when you complete it. Go into another cross-legged crouch, this time with your *right* knee over your left.

Pivot on your feet and turn to the *left*, making another 360-degree turn, and go into another crouch, now with your left knee over your right.

Practice these pivoting turns and crouches until you've got them. You're doing great.

(continued)

HALF-CROSSED SEATED STANCE (cont.)

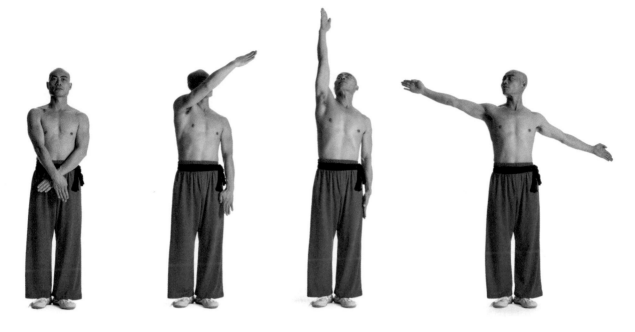

Now learn to do the arm rotation, head turns, and strike without using your legs. Stand straight and relaxed, feet together. With your palms flat, cross your wrists over your groin like you're protecting your privates. In Chinese this is described as "*Shizi cha zhang hu dang qian*" (十字插掌護襠前). You can start in either direction, but for this example begin with your right wrist crossed on top of your left.

Rotate your arms *clockwise*. Remember to fully extend your arms and whole body. When you're training, you're also stretching, and you'll feel it down to your toes. Lead with your right hand, raising it from your groin in a flat arc across your chest and then up past your left shoulder. When your right arm is almost straight up beside your head, begin to follow with your left arm, rotating out in a flat arc to your left side. Continue rotating your right arm up over your head, and then down, until your arm is down at your right side. Simultaneously, your left arm rotates straight up beside your head, fingertips pointed to the sky. If you were a clock, your arms would be pointing to 6 o'clock:

your right hand pointing down at the 6, your left hand up at the 12.

Continue to rotate your arms and bend your elbows to bring your forearms together in front of your navel, your left forearm on top of the right, your right palm facing up, left palm down.

Understand? Practice this arm rotation several times until you've got it.

Go back to the start and add the head turns. Rotate your arms. As you rotate your arms, your head follows your right palm. Turn your head to the left as your right palm rotates up past your left shoulder, and then to the right as your right arm rotates down to your right side. Keep your head facing right as you bring your arms together in front of you.

Now for the strike. You're going to strike to the *left* with your left palm. Rotate your arms and bring them together in front of your navel like you've just been practicing.

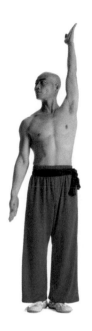 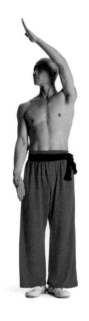 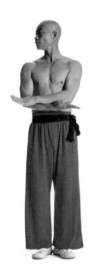 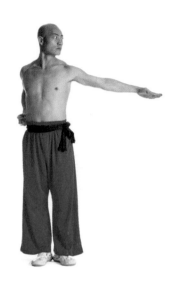

Remember to turn your head to the left, and then to the right, so that your face is turned right as you bring your arms together in front of you. Strike out quickly with your left palm to your left side, like a blade slicing through the air, with your palm down and your arm at about a 45-degree angle to the ground. At the exact same time, snap your head to the left and simultaneously chamber your right fist. Pow!

When you strike, make sure your arm is fully extended out to your side. Don't let it go back behind you. From your right shoulder to your left fingers should be one straight line—just like you should be straightforward in life, not living snake-style!

Also, when you strike to the left and chamber your right fist, pull your right shoulder back, opening your chest wide. This is using the power of opposites so you strike with explosive power. Bam!

Practice this arm rotation and left strike several times until you can do it smoothly and swiftly. Got it? Great!

Now practice striking to the right. It's exactly the reverse. Cross your wrists over your groin, left wrist on top of right. Rotate your arms *counterclockwise*, leading with the left, and bring your forearms together in front of your navel with your right forearm crossed on top of your left, right palm down, left palm up. As you rotate your arms, your head follows your left palm, turning first to the right and then to the left. Strike quickly to the right with your right palm, and at the same time chamber your left fist while snapping your head to the right. Make sure your right arm is fully extended to your side. Don't let it go back behind you. And remember to use the power of opposites, pulling your left shoulder back when you strike and opening your chest wide when you strike—bam!

Understand? Practice alternating these right and left strikes. Do them 10 times. *Yi*—right strike. *Er*—left strike. *San*—right strike. *Si*—left strike. . . .

Fantastic.

(continued)

HALF-CROSSED SEATED STANCE (cont.)

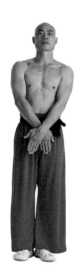 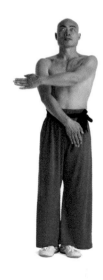 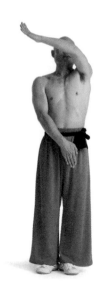 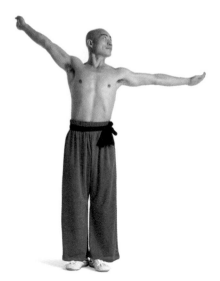

The next step is to combine the arms, legs, body, and head into one movement. Let's strike to the right first.

Stand straight and relaxed, feet together, wrists crossed in front of your groin, left wrist on top of right. Rotate your arms counterclockwise and bend your elbows to bring your forearms together in front of your navel, right arm on top of left, right palm facing down, left palm facing up. Don't forget to follow your left arm with your head, turning your head to the right and then to the left. When you bring your arms together in front of your navel, lift your left foot. At the exact same time that you plant your left foot in front of the right and bend your knees into a crossed-legged crouch, strike to the right, chambering your left fist and snapping your head to the right. Pow!

Understand? Practice this cross-legged Xie Bu strike to the right several times until your body understands it.

You look magnificent.

Let's continue. You've struck to the right. Now you're going to pivot and strike to the left. Here's how to do it.

Execute the cross-legged crouch and strike to the right. Now pivot on your feet to turn your body to the right, making a

360-degree turn so that you're facing front again when you complete it (see photos on pages 180 and 181). At the exact same time that you begin to pivot and turn your body, begin to rotate your arms. You rotate them *clockwise*, with the right arm leading. Remember also to turn your head, following your right arm first to the left and then to the right.

At the halfway point—where you have pivoted and turned 180 degrees—your arms should be extended straight out to your sides from your shoulders. At this point in the arm rotation, begin to make a small circle with your right arm so that your right palm turns from facing down to facing up.

Continue to pivot and turn your body, coming around the full 360 degrees to face the way you started out. Notice that as you complete the turn, your right foot is in front of your left.

As you complete the turn, you're also completing the arm rotation, bending your elbows to bring your forearms together in front of your navel, left arm on top of the right, with the left palm facing down and the right palm facing up. When you bring your arms together, learn the movement known as Shaolin Qin Na (擒拿), which means "capturing," or "grappling," an attacker's arm or wrist between your own.

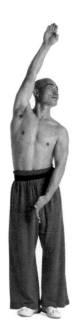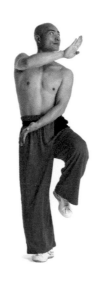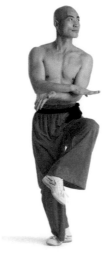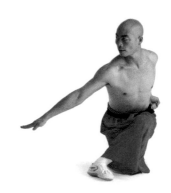

Here's how you do it: When you are bringing your arms together, imagine that you've caught an opponent's wrist between your arms. As you complete the turn and go into the cross-legged crouch, continue to turn your crossed arms and your upper body farther to the right, as though you're pulling the attacker's arm down, to the right and into your body, using your body's weight and power—which would be very painful for him, as well as pull him off balance.

And now strike, extending your left palm quickly to the side like a blade, at the same time that you chamber your right fist and snap your head to the left. All movements should be completed at exactly the same moment, in one explosion of power—the cross-legged crouch, the left strike, the chambering of your right fist, and the left head snap. Bam! Your attacker, whose arm you captured with Qin Na before you struck him with your left palm, is hitting the ground!

Understand? Practice the whole sequence of moves from the beginning. Execute a cross-legged crouch and strike to the right. Then pivot on your feet to turn 360 degrees, rotating your arms and bringing them together in front of your navel as you turn. As you complete the turn and go into another cross-legged crouch, right foot in front of left, add the Qin Na grappling movement with your body and arms, and then strike to the left. Pow!

Got it? Fantastic!

After the left strike, you can turn around and strike to the right again. Just reverse the direction. Turn and pivot to the left 360 degrees, rotating your arms *counterclockwise*, with your left arm leading. Remember to follow your left hand with your head, turning it right, then left. As you're completing the turn and assuming the cross-legged crouch (now with your left foot in front of the right), bring your forearms together with your right arm on top of your left, do the Qin Na grappling move, and then strike to the right. Bam!

Practice these Xie Bu turns and strikes until you understand them. Strike right, pivot and turn, strike left, pivot and turn in the opposite direction, strike right again . . . and so on.

Beautiful! You look like a true Shaolin warrior.

As you keep practicing Xie Bu over the coming days, you'll learn to do it with speed and fluidity, completing each turn with an explosive strike. It's a beautiful and powerful move, and it's great for developing your balance, coordination, and strength. You'll love the feeling of confidence you get from mastering it.

(continued)

HALF-CROSSED SEATED STANCE (cont.)

From Right Strike to Left Strike

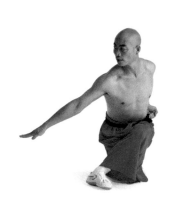 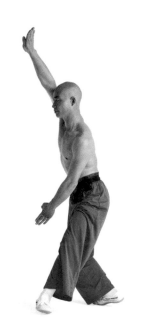 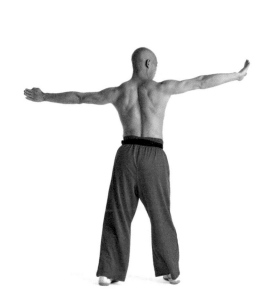

From Left Strike to Right Strike

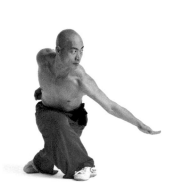 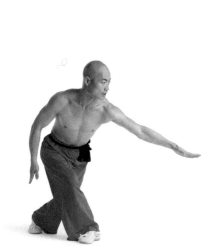 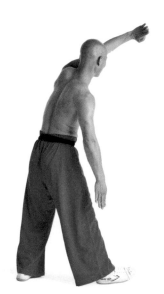

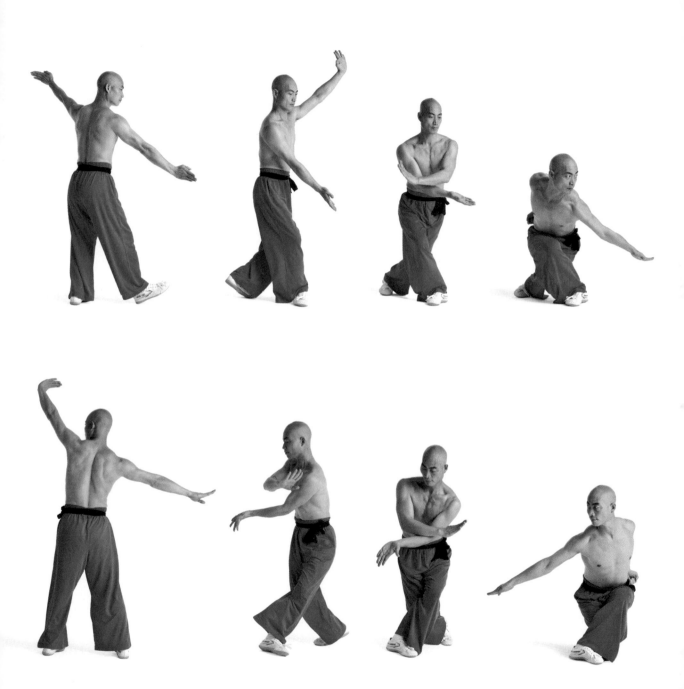

Meditation

Confidence is the key to success.

Sifu wants you to be able to defend yourself and protect others if the need ever arises. But he does not teach any of his students the fight applications of these movements, because he doesn't want you to be limited in your mind. We learn kung fu to free our minds from too much thinking. That's why he always tells you, "Don't think. Just do it." If you were ever in a real fight situation where you had to defend yourself or someone else, if you thought too much, you would lose. Once you've begun to think, you've already lost the fight. In a real fight, you must react quickly, instinctively, and with complete confidence.

At Shaolin Temple, Sifu was taught that there are four keys to success in a real fight. In order of importance, they are:

Dan ("confidence")
Duan ("a short time")
Ji ("skills")
Shan ("movement")

Notice that *dan*, confidence, is the first and most important. If you don't have confidence in yourself, don't fight, because you will surely be beaten by your more confident opponent, even if he has no *ji*.

Next in importance is *duan*, to act in a short time, with speed. From speed comes power. Don't stand there thinking about it—act quickly, with complete confidence.

Ji, skills, comes only third in importance. If you don't have *dan* and *duan*—confidence and quickness—your handsome form, harmonies, and knowledge mean nothing.

Last is *shan*, movement. If you don't have *dan*, *duan*, and *ji*, move—run away!

As with everything else in kung fu training, this lesson can be applied to your entire life. Confidence is the most important key to success in all areas of your life. Believe in yourself. Trust yourself. If you lack self-confidence, you can't get the job done. You will find it difficult to succeed in any endeavor. You will let the obstacles, problems, and tasks your life throws at you defeat you.

Face your day today with the confidence that you can handle any task, solve any problem, and overcome any obstacle.

"AMITUOFO! AMITUOFO! AMITUOFO!"

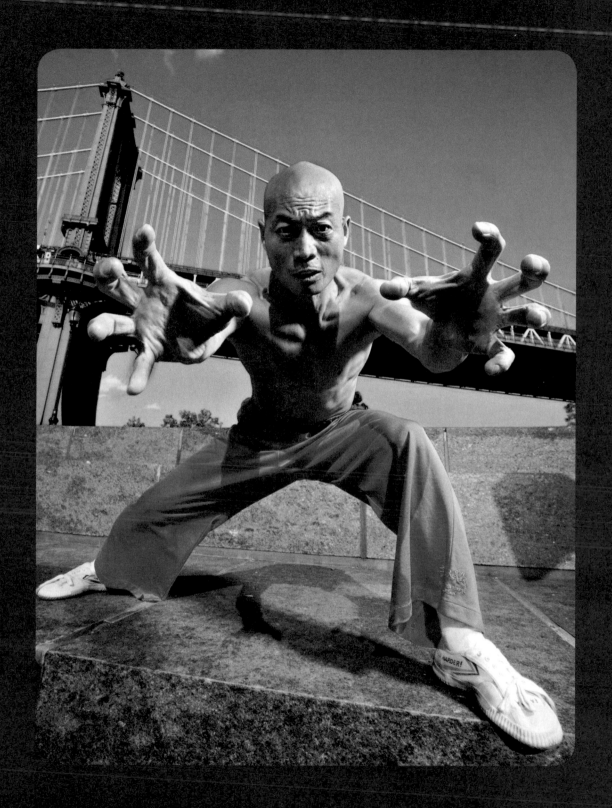

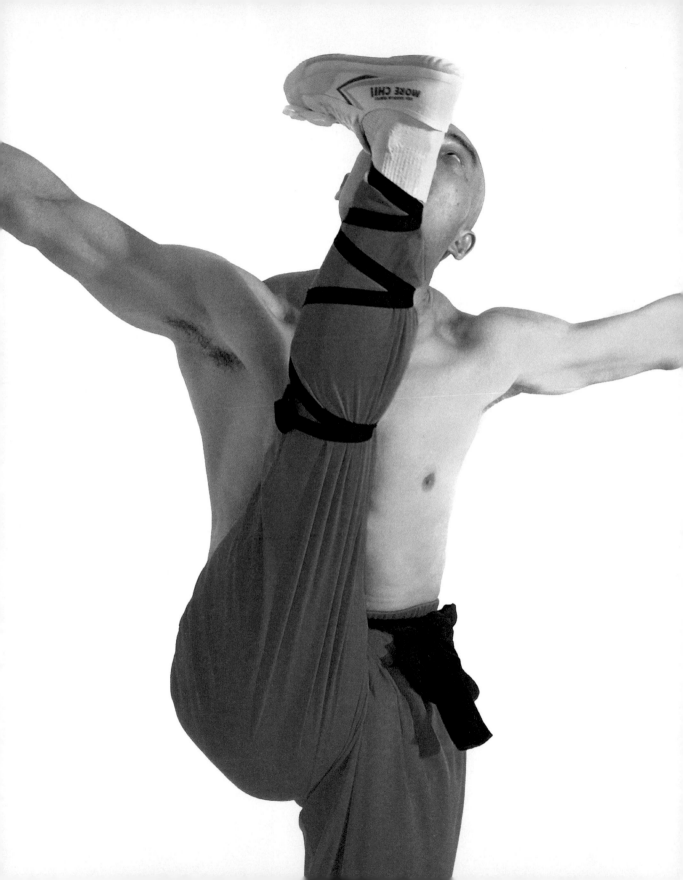

Front Flex Kick

"AMITUOFO!"
"AMITUOFO!"
"AMITUOFO!"

Begin as usual, going through your entire routine,
from wrist rotations straight up through Xie Bu.

FRONT FLEX KICK
(Zhengtitui)

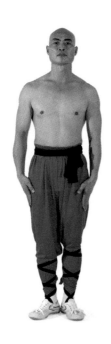
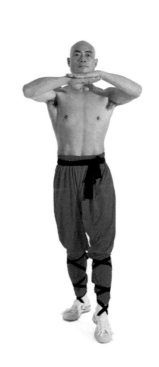
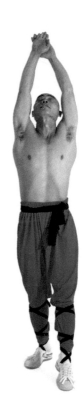

Zhengtitui (pronounced *jung-tee-twee*) should be relatively simple to learn, because it doesn't have so many "moving parts." That doesn't mean it can instantly be mastered! When you master this kick, you will be able to do it with such precision that you can vary the points of your head that your toes touch, kicking your forehead, your nose, your chin, or your ear as you wish. You'll be able to answer the cell phone without using your hands—no kidding!

To begin, break it down into separate elements.

Stand straight and relaxed, fully extended, feet together.

Yu bei! To go into the ready position, combine arms and legs simultaneously. Quickly lift your arms together in front of you, elbows bent, and slap your palms together in front of your chin. Do not swing your arms out to your sides and then back in—lift them in front of you. As you slap your palms, take a small step forward with one foot—let's make it the left for this example—onto your toes. Fully extend your entire body when you do this, from the tips of your toes to the top of your head. Pop your body!

The next move uses only your arms and head. First, lift your arms straight up, close to your head, palms forward, fingers pointing to the sky, and cross your hands. Follow your right hand with your head and look up.

Now quickly lower your arms out to your sides and slightly back at shoulder height, throwing your chest

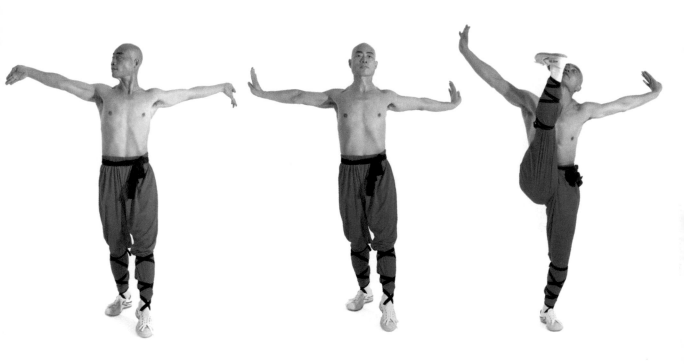

open and out, and snap your palms down like blades cutting the terrible things from your life, while you snap your head to the right.

Now snap your palms up so that they are facing straight out to the left and right and your fingers are pointing up, at the same time that you snap your head to look forward. See the dolphins dancing in front of you.

You will maintain your arms in this position through the rest of the kick.

Practice executing this series of arm, palm, and head movements a few times, doing them quickly and sharply. Snap! Snap! Snap! You'll be using the same

movements when you learn the kicks called Lihetui and Waibaitui.

Now for the kick.

Zou! Take a small step forward with your left foot, planting it flat on the ground. Kick straight up toward your head with your right leg, toes flexed, both knees locked. Keep your legs and your body fully extended when you kick. Don't bend your legs, and don't bend or lean your body forward into the kick. Keep your body fully extended and your chest open, like you're offering your loving heart to the world. Also, don't drop your arms or bend them like you're surrendering! Keep them fully extended straight out from the shoulders to the sides.

(continued)

FRONT FLEX KICK (cont.)

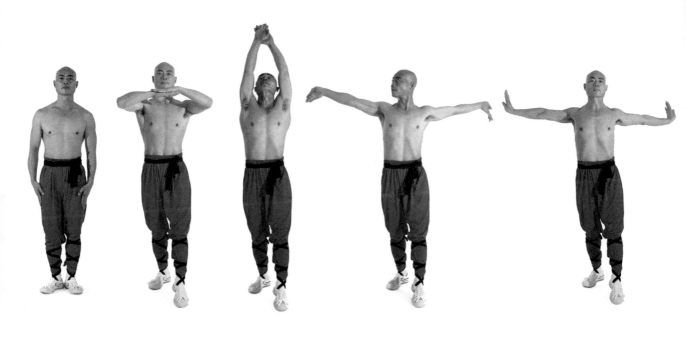

Hold your hips in when you kick, to aim your foot toward your head. Don't open your hips or kick out to the side.

Kick your chin, and at that instant point your toes for landing and fully extend your body even higher. Lower your leg with the same speed that you kicked up. Kick up and down quick as lightning, expressing an explosive whip crack of chi at the top of the kick, and land on your toes, light as a leaf.

Understand? Practice this right kick until your body gets it, from the starting position to landing on your toes.

Gorgeous!

When you complete a right kick, you can step directly into a left kick. When your right foot lands on its toes, take a small step forward with that foot, and kick up toward your head with your left leg. Remember to keep your whole body fully extended from your toes to your head, both knees locked, and your arms fully extended to the sides and a little behind your shoulders. When your left foot lands on its toes, take a small step forward with that foot and then kick up with your right leg. And so on, kick-marching toward the dolphins.

Practice this now. Kick right, take a small step; kick left, small step; kick right . . .

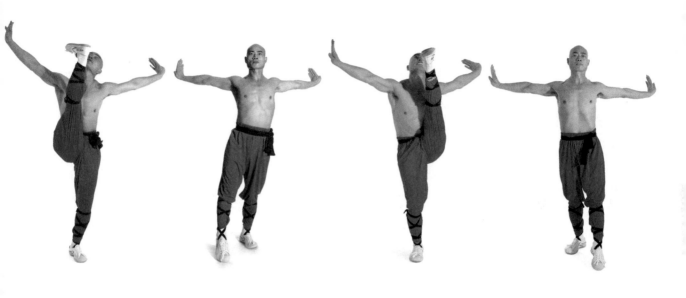

Brilliant. You can practice Zhengtitui in different versions. If you want to practice the kicks without the arms at first, fold your arms behind you, throw open your chest, and kick. Or you can lay a pole, a broom, or a mop across your shoulders behind your neck and hold it there with your hands.

Also, in a small space you can practice a stationary version. Kick with your right foot and land it lightly on its toes, and then kick with your left foot, and so on, without moving forward. You can do this holding on to something beside you for support—a wall, a tree, a stretching bar, a porch railing, a backyard fence. You can train everywhere, because the temple is everywhere.

Feel it working your entire body—your legs, buttocks, back, hips, groin muscles, chest, arms, shoulders, neck, head. Don't worry if you don't reach your head with your toes today. You will. Every day that you train, you'll kick a little higher. Believe in yourself. Trust yourself. Have confidence in yourself.

Meditation

*Life is sometimes bitter, sometimes spicy, sometimes sour, sometimes sweet.
But it is always beautiful.*

When Da Mo accepted Shen Guang as his disciple, he took him up Drum Mountain, in front of Shaolin Temple and below Shao-shu Mountain. It's called Drum Mountain because of its flat top. Da Mo dug him a well so he would have water to drink, cook, and bathe with, and instructed him to stay up there, meditating, for 1 year.

The water of the well was bitter, but Shen Guang endured it for a year. Then he came down and asked Da Mo, "What's next?" Da Mo took him back up Drum Mountain and dug him a second well. The water of this well was spicy. Shen Guang endured.

At the end of the second year, Shen Guang came to Da Mo and asked, "What's next?" Da Mo took him back up the mountain and dug him a third well. This time the water was sour.

A year later, Shen Guang came to Da Mo and asked, "What's next?" Da Mo took him back up the mountain and dug a fourth well. This time the water was sweet.

At that point Shen Guang realized the lesson Da Mo was teaching him. Without speaking, Da Mo had told him everything. When you begin to speak, you can't stop talking. Remind yourself to talk less and do more!

Here's what Shen Guang understood Da Mo was teaching him: Life is like the water in those wells. Sometimes it's bitter, sometimes it's spicy, sometimes it's sour, and sometimes it's sweet. In Chinese that's *ku* ("bitter"), *la* ("spicy"), *suan* ("sour"), *tian* ("sweet"). It's like the four seasons: *chun* ("spring"), *xia* ("summer"), *qiu* ("fall"), *dong* ("winter"). That's part of the beauty of life, that it is always changing, always moving. Think how dull and tedious life would be if all you ever had to eat was just herbs or just curry or just salt or just sugar. Or if every single day the weather were exactly the same as yesterday's and tomorrow's. Think of how dull *you* would be if you never changed, never grew, never moved, never faced a new challenge, just remained a lump of a person from birth until death!

Learn to appreciate the change and richness that is life, in all its moods, all its flavors, all kinds of weather. Some days life seems easy and good; some days it seems very hard to endure. Some days it's sunny and springlike; some days it's hot and summery; some days it's cool and fall-like; some days it's wintry and cold. One day you break up with someone you love, and then you meet and fall in love with someone new.

Whether it's bitter, spicy, sour, or sweet, life is always a beautiful gift. You can appreciate it in all its diversity if you keep your heart flat, like the top of Drum Mountain.

"AMITUOFO! AMITUOFO! AMITUOFO!"

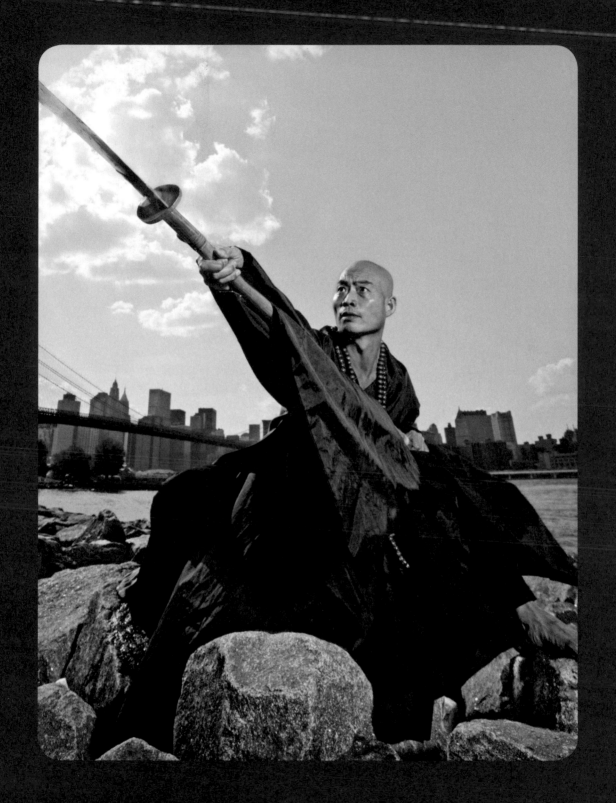

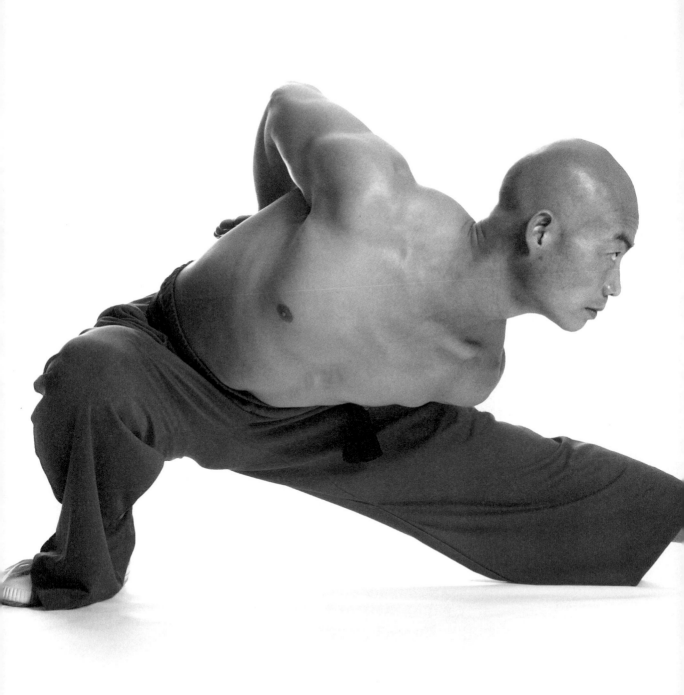

Crouched Stance

"AMITUOFO!"
"AMITUOFO!"
"AMITUOFO!"

To begin, work through your entire routine as usual.

CROUCHED STANCE
(Pu Bu)

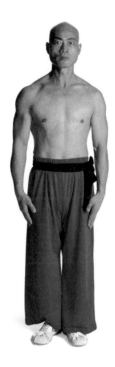
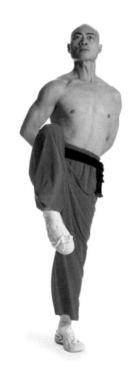
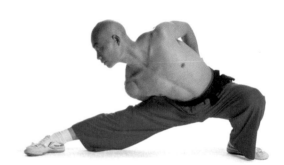

Pu Bu (pronounced *poo boo*) is a graphic reminder of why you've been repeating and repeating your stretches to increase your flexibility. It's built directly on the Pu Bu Yatui stretches you've been practicing.

To begin, break it down into its elements, starting with the legs.

Stand straight and relaxed, fully extended. Because you won't be using your arms yet, just fold them behind you. You can begin with either foot; for this example, let's make it the right foot.

Bend your knee and lift your right leg in front of you as high and fast as you comfortably can, foot extended and toes pointing down.

Now execute a Pu Bu stance to the right. Quickly extend the right leg out to the side, knee locked, planting the right foot flat, right toes pointing straight ahead. At the same time, crouch with the left leg, bending the left knee and lowering yourself until your left thigh is parallel to the ground. Your left foot should be pointing 45 degrees to the left. Don't go down so low that you're resting the back of your thigh on your lower leg—that's cheating. Go down

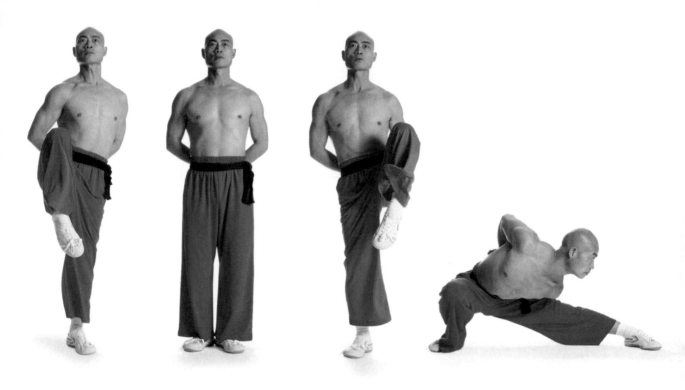

only until your left thigh is parallel to the ground. Keep that left foot firmly planted flat on the ground.

As you go down into the Pu Bu stance, lean your body toward your extended right leg. Fully extend your body. Don't curl your back, don't lean forward, and don't lean to the opposite side. Extend your body as far as you can to the right while maintaining your balance.

Now you're going to go directly into a Pu Bu in the opposite direction. Come back up to center, your original position, from the right Pu Bu, lifting your right foot and

putting your legs together. Stand with your body fully extended, lift your left leg as high and quickly as you comfortably can, and execute a Pu Bu to the left.

From there, come back up to center, legs together, and go instantly into a right Pu Bu. Then come up to center and go into one to the left. And so on, alternating side to side.

Practice this alternating sequence 10 times. *Yi*—right. *Er*—left. *San*—right . . .

Got it? Very good.

(continued)

CROUCHED STANCE (cont.)

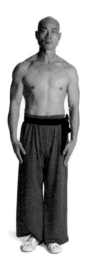 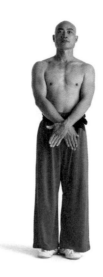 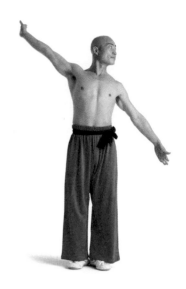

Add arm rotations and strikes.

Stand straight and relaxed, fully extended, and cross your wrists in front of your groin, palms flat, the same as you do in Xie Bu. You will be striking to the right for this example, so cross your left wrist over your right one.

Rotate your arms *counterclockwise*, just as you do in Xie Bu: Lead with your left hand, swinging it in a wide arc up over your head and down to the left side. Meanwhile, your right arm follows up over your head. Your arms are at

6 o'clock, left hand pointing to the 6, right hand to the 12. Don't forget to follow your left hand with your head, turning right and then left.

As you complete the arm rotations, bend your elbows to bring your forearms together in front of your navel, right arm on top of the left, right palm down, left palm up. Simultaneously, lift your right foot and go into your Pu Bu to the right. As you plant your right foot, strike to the right with your right palm while chambering your left fist. Extend your right arm and your upper body as fully as you can to

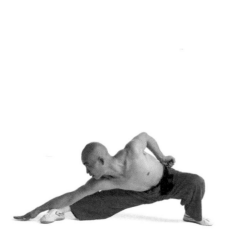 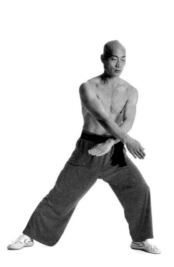 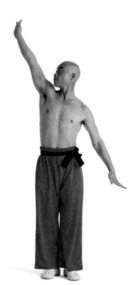

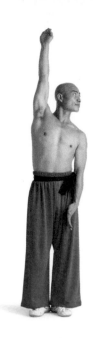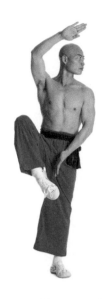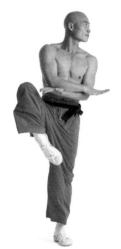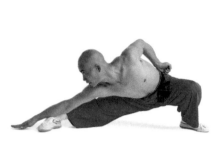

the right when you strike. Your goal is to extend so far that your right hand strikes out over your extended right foot. Also, remember to pull your left shoulder back when you chamber your fist, popping your chest open and using the power of opposites to give the strike extra chi. Bam!

Practice this right strike until you understand.

Got it? Marvelous. Continue. Follow the right strike with one to the left, simply reversing direction. Here's how to do it.

Execute a Pu Bu strike to the right. Then, as you come up out of it, simultaneously begin to rotate your arms *clockwise* this time, leading with your right arm. Follow your right hand with your head, first to the left and then to the right. Your legs, arms, and head move at the same time and in total harmony. As you bring your forearms together in front of your navel, lift your left foot as high and as quickly as you comfortably can and execute a Pu Bu to the left. As you plant your left foot, strike with your left palm and chamber your right fist. Pow!

(continued)

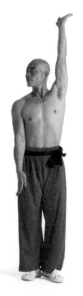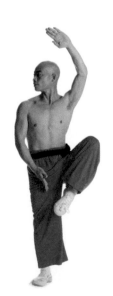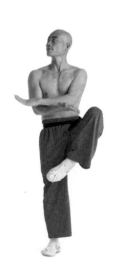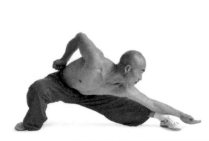

CROUCHED STANCE (cont.)

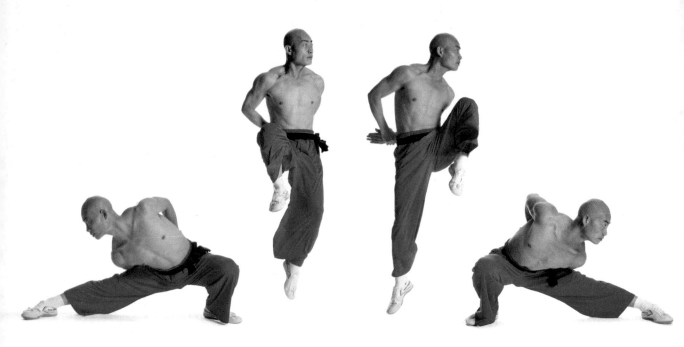

Understand? And now you can come up out of that left strike and strike to the right again. And so on, alternating left and right.

Practice alternating these right and left Pu Bu strikes until your body understands them. Add more speed

and chi with each repetition. Strike right—pow! Strike left—bam! You look awesome.

Now add one more element to the sequence—a hop jump. Practice it first with just the legs, no arm rotations or strikes. Fold your arms behind your back.

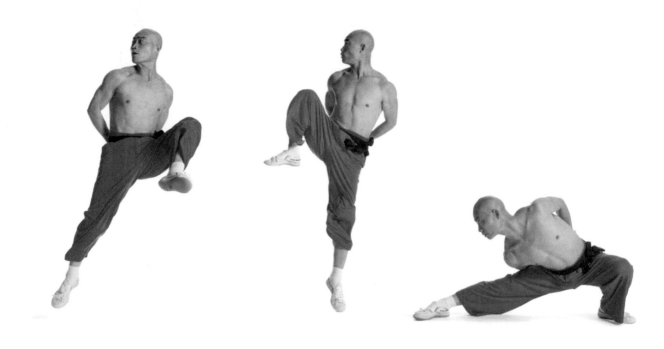

Execute a Pu Bu stance to the right. Now, instead of merely rising and going into a left Pu Bu, *hop* up off your right foot as high and as quickly as you comfortably can and, at almost the same instant, lift your left leg as high and as quickly as you comfortably can. For a second your body will be in the air, both feet off the ground. Extend your left leg to your left as you go down into a left Pu Bu. And hey—don't forget to fully extend your upper body. Reach for the sky when you hop-jump.

Try it, practicing this hop jump until your body understands.

(continued)

CROUCHED STANCE (cont.)

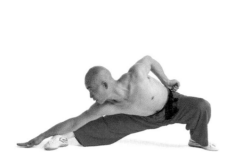

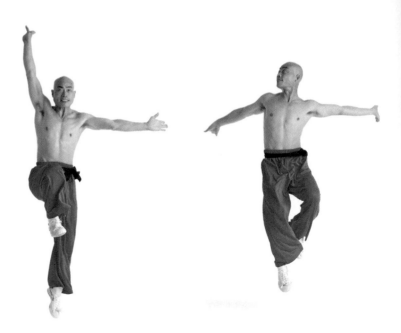

Now add the arm rotations and strikes. Execute a Pu Bu strike to the right. Now, as you hop up off your right foot, rotate your arms *clockwise*, leading with your right arm, and come down into a left strike. Remember to follow your right hand with your head, turning it left and then right. Then snap your head to the left when you do the left strike.

Your legs, arms, and head should all move at the same time and in perfect harmony, beginning and ending their moves exactly together.

Practice this right strike/hop jump/left strike sequence until you understand it. Your arms and legs may get a bit confused at first, but keep practicing and you'll find yourself getting better at it with every repetition.

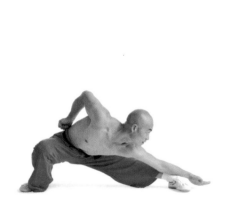

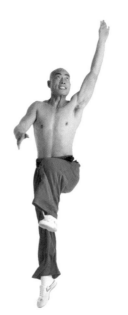

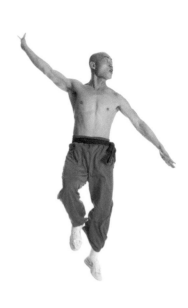

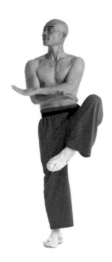

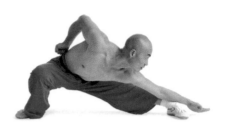

Got it? Bravo! Now that you understand the sequence, you can keep alternating right and left Pu Bu strikes as long as you like. They're simply the reverse of each other. Execute a Pu Bu strike to the right, hop-jump up and execute a Pu Bu to the left, hop-jump and execute a Pu Bu to the right, and so on.

Try doing it 10 times in a row, alternating right and left. *Yi*—strike right. *Er*—strike left. *San*—strike right. *Si*—strike left. . . . Add speed and power with each repetition until you're executing your Pu Bu hop jumps and strikes like a fearsome kung fu warrior, leaping off the ground with the ferocity of a tiger. Fabulous!

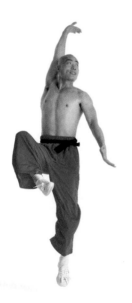

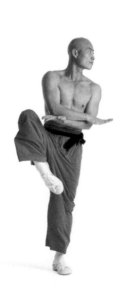

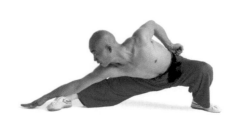

Meditation

I can't love others if I don't love myself. I can't expect others to respect me if I don't respect myself.

Kung fu isn't just an exercise routine. It is a philosophy of life. The action is the philosophy. The philosophy is the action. The two are inseparable, just as the head and body cannot be separated and live.

Through kung fu you're learning mental and physical discipline. You're beginning to develop a beautiful mind in a beautiful body. You're polishing your body and your mind to polish your life, the better to express your inner and outer beauty. In mastering your body and your mind, you will master your life. In respecting your body, you learn to respect yourself. You can't expect others to respect you if you don't respect yourself. You can't love others if you don't love yourself.

"AMITUOFO! AMITUOFO! AMITUOFO!"

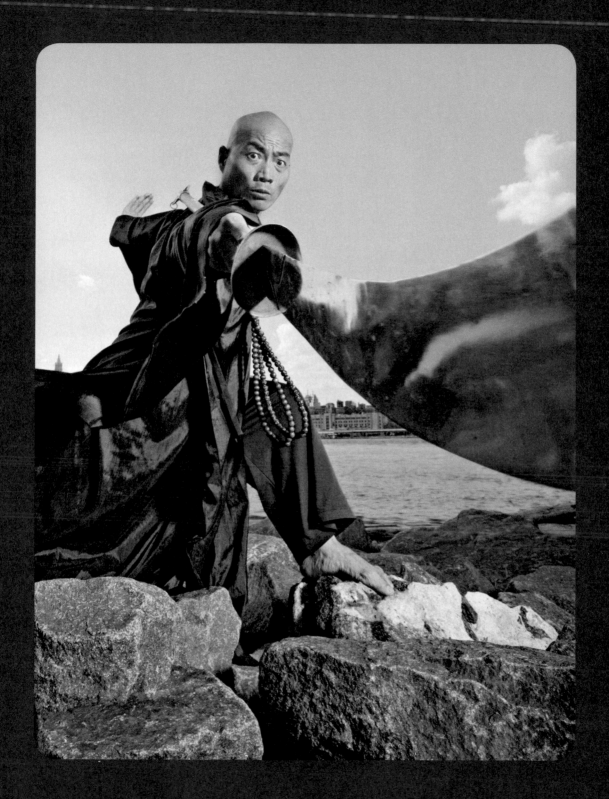

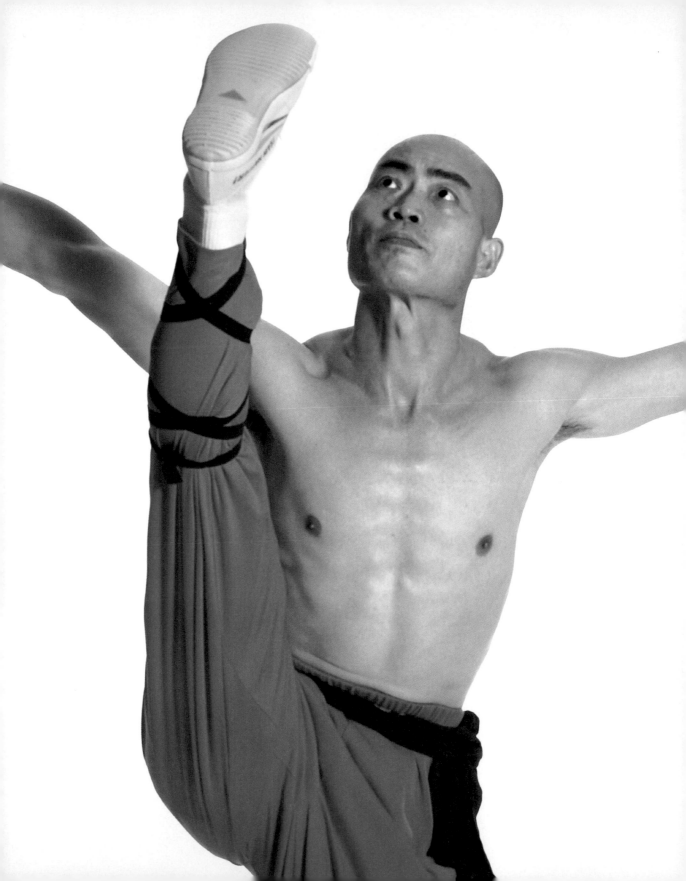

Inside Crescent Kick

"AMITUOFO!"
"AMITUOFO!"
"AMITUOFO!"

Begin with your usual routine, all the way up through Pu Bu.

Notice how the first stances and kicks you practiced have become much more natural and fluid with daily training. Keep increasing your speed and extension as you execute them. Kick a little higher today. Extend a little farther. Put more chi into your entire routine!

INSIDE CRESCENT KICK
(Lihetui)

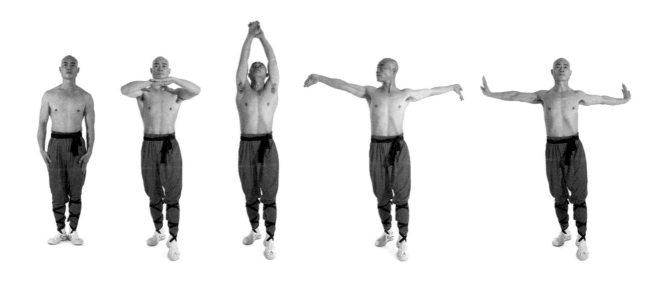

Lihetui (pronounced *lee-huh-twee*) is an inside crescent kick, because you kick your leg out in an arc from the hip and then up toward your face.

Learn it in steps.

Stand straight and relaxed, fully extended, feet together. Now, exactly as you've been doing in Zhengtitui, quickly lift your arms together in front of you, elbows bent, and slap your palms together in front of your chin, at the same time that you take a small step forward with one foot—let's make it the left for this example—and land on your toes. Fully extend your entire body when you do this, from the tips of your toes to the top of your head. Remem-

ber, don't swing your arms out to your sides and back in when you lift them. Lift them straight up in front of you and slap your palms.

Then lift your arms straight up, close to your head, palms forward, fingers pointing to the sky, and cross your hands. Follow your right hand with your head and look up.

Quickly lower your arms to your sides and slightly back at shoulder height, and snap your palms down like blades while you snap your head to the right.

Snap your palms up so that they are facing straight out to the left and right and your fingers are pointing up, at

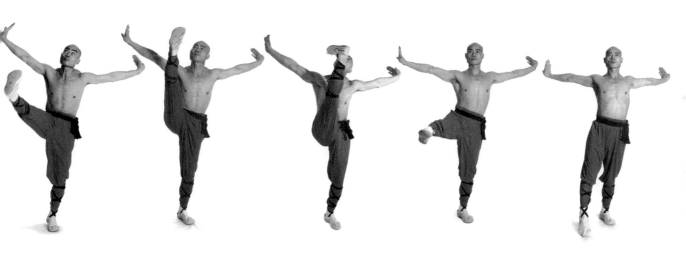

the same time that you snap your head to look forward. See your beautiful future ahead of you. You will maintain your arms in this position through the rest of the kick.

Now kick with your right leg fully extended, your knee locked, and your right foot flexed to aim your toes toward your head. Do not kick straight up. Kick from the outside in, about 45 degrees out to the right and then back in toward your face. Kick close to your face. Sifu says make it a new rule: When you wash your face, never use your hands—use your feet! When you kick close to your face, express an explosion of chi, point your toes for landing, and extend your body up higher—pop it!

Then lower your leg straight down the center as quickly as it kicked up, landing soft as a feather on your toes in front of you.

Understand? Practice it. Remember to flex your foot as you kick your leg up, and then extend your foot and point your toes as it comes down. Keep your whole body fully extended as you kick. Don't bend your knees or lean your body forward. As you kick, don't turn your body or watch your foot—keep your body straight and fully extended, with your eyes looking straight ahead. Don't drop or bend your arms, either.

You look amazing!

(continued)

INSIDE CRESCENT KICK (cont.)

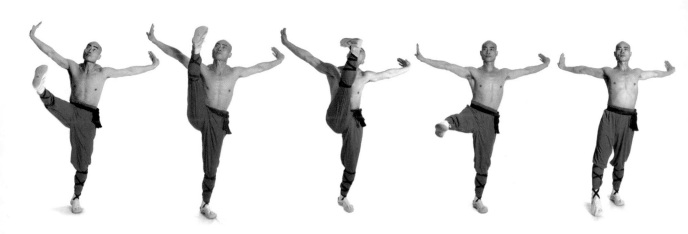

Now learn to travel, alternating right and left kicks. Execute a right kick. When your right foot lands on its toes, take a small step forward with your right foot, and then kick up with the left. Kick from the outside in, toward your face. Wash your face with your foot! When your foot is closest to your face, extend the toes for landing and extend your body upward. Land your left foot on its toes; then take a small step with that foot and kick up with the right. And so on, marching toward your beautiful future.

Practice this now, traveling 10 kicks forward. *Yi*—right kick. *Er*—left kick. *San*—right kick....

If you're training in a small space, you can also alternate right and left kicks standing in one place. Execute a right

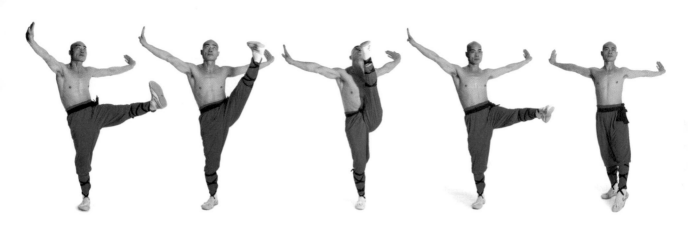

kick, land that foot on its toes, and then execute a left kick without taking a step forward in between. You can also use a wall, a tree, a stretching bar, a railing, or a fence for support while you learn.

Fabulous. Don't worry if you can't kick as high as your face today. Keep training every day, and your kicks will keep getting a little higher. Remember, don't cheat by leaning forward. Keep your body fully extended. Reach for your face with your feet. Soon you'll be able to kick so high that you can wash your face with your feet. And then, with continued practice, you'll be kicking *higher*. No question!

Meditation

Beautiful birds always land on the top of the tree.
Brilliant people always express their journeys up higher.

Have you ever seen a "lazy" bird? There's no such thing. Birds are constantly active, constantly expressing their beautiful lives in their songs, their bright feathers, their soaring flight overhead. Birds are bursting with chi! And they don't have time to waste being lazy. If a bird were too lazy to fly, to hunt, to sing, it would never find a meal or a mate.

Physical laziness, mental laziness, and spiritual laziness reinforce one another. When your body has no energy, your mind is dull. You have no chi. Your life is like water running downhill. You waste so much time just lying around, no energy to move, no interest in anything. And then, before you know it, you run out of time to waste.

No one really wants to live that way. Watch the birds overhead. Watch them soaring, arcing, zipping across the sky. And then observe where they land. The beautiful birds always land first at the top of the tree.

In your life, you should be reaching for the top as well. Don't be like water running downhill. Be like the beautiful birds, exploding with chi, soaring, singing, spreading their colorful wings. Express yourself through your body. Express your beauty, inside and out. Live your whole day with the same level of dedication, focus, and energy you're putting into your Shaolin Workout. Apply the cheer of "More chi!" not just to your workout sessions but to your whole life.

"AMITUOFO! AMITUOFO! AMITUOFO!"

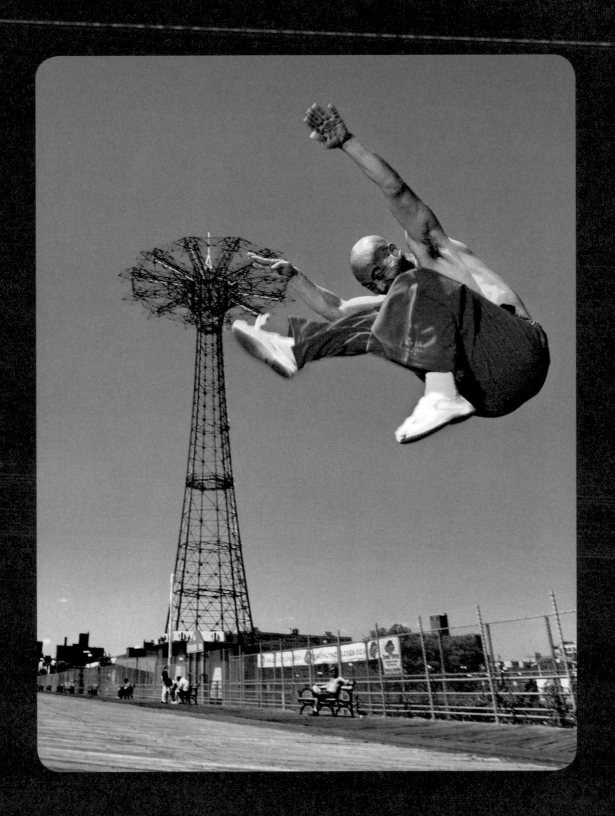

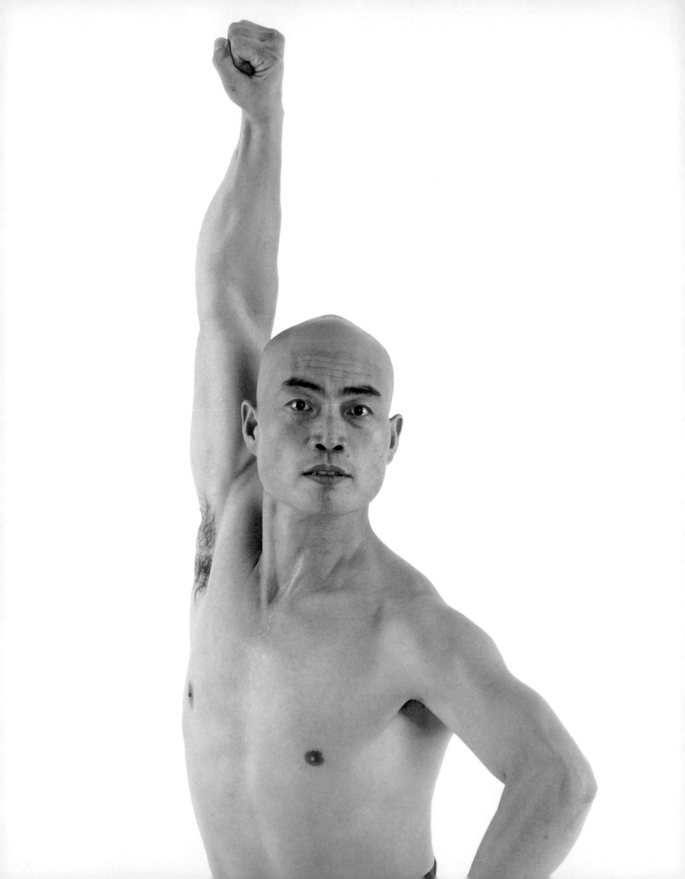

Hollow Stance

"AMITUOFO!"
"AMITUOFO!"
"AMITUOFO!"

First, complete your entire routine, up through Lihetui. More chi! Train harder!

HOLLOW STANCE
(Xu Bu)

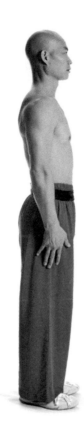

Xu Bu (pronounced *shoo boo*) is called the hollow stance, because your back leg carries all your weight and power, while your front leg is weightless, as if it were hollow. It's a crouched, traveling stance that enhances your balance, coordination, and harmonies.

Let's break the stance down to its elements, starting with the legs.

Stand straight and relaxed, fully extended.

Now bend both knees so that you are in a comfortable crouch, almost like you're sitting in an invisible chair. Stay in that "seated" crouch and take a small step forward with one foot—let's make it the left foot for this example—and bring that foot down on its toes. There should be no weight placed on your left foot, no power—again, as though that leg were hollow. All the weight and power are in your right leg. Be mindful not to lean forward—keep your back straight and fully extended.

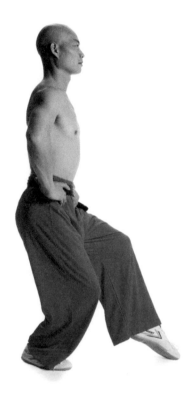

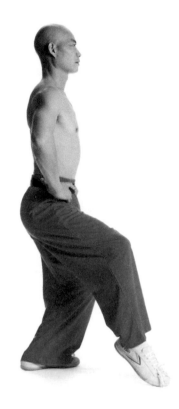

Now you're going to crouch-walk forward. Your body should maintain the same height throughout the following movements. Don't rise by straightening your knees. Keep the knees bent so you remain in the seated crouch throughout. Step forward with the right foot onto its toes as you plant the left foot flat. Then just keep traveling. Take a small step forward with your left foot, stepping onto its toes, then the right, then the left, moving forward toward the dolphins. Don't come up out of the seated crouch at any point. As always, keep your body

fully extended, head and chin up, shoulders square. Remember that each time you step forward, you plant the back foot flat on the ground.

Practice these traveling Xu Bu steps until your body understands them.

Excellent. Now add the next element—arm rotations with a pivoting turn. You will learn two versions: one for palms, the other for fists.

(continued)

HOLLOW STANCE (cont.)

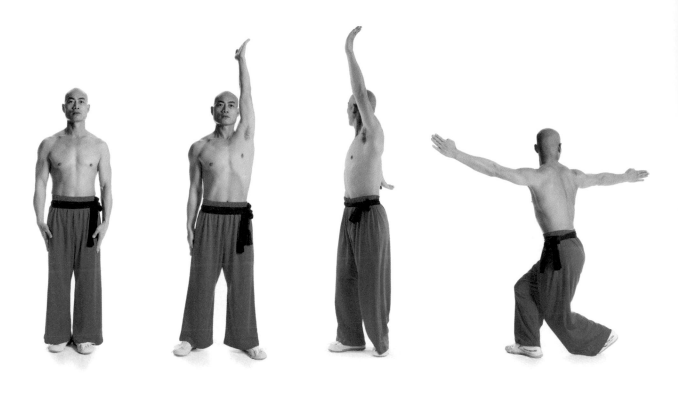

Begin with the palm version. Stand straight and relaxed, fully extended. Lift your left arm straight above your head, palm forward, fingers pointing to the sky, and place your right arm straight down to your side, fingers pointing to the ground. Your arms are in the 6 o'clock position, with your left hand pointing to the 12 and your right hand pointing to the 6.

Now you're going to use the arm rotations you've been practicing since all the way back in Session 3. As you begin to rotate your arms—the left arm forward and down, the right arm back and up— follow your right arm with your head, turning it to the right. Simultaneously, bend your knees and turn your body to the right, pivoting on your right foot. Do not take a step; just pivot. Execute all these actions simultaneously, so you begin rotating your arms,

turning your body and head, and bending your knees all in harmony.

Continue rotating your arms. When your right palm is above your head, snap your palm so that it is facing out to the right and your fingers are pointed forward at about a 45-degree angle. Keep a very slight bend in that elbow—don't overextend it. Don't bend your wrist. At the same time, snap your head and turn your body to face forward, pivoting on the right foot as you take a small step forward with the left foot onto its toes. As you take that step, place your left palm on your upper thigh, with the thumb on the outside of your thigh and the fingers on the inside. Complete all of these actions simultaneously and in full harmony.

Understand? Practice these arm rotations, body and head turns, and one step forward with your

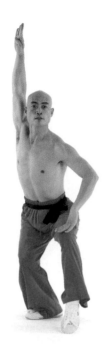 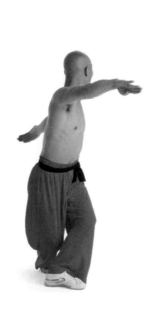 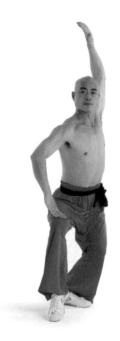

left foot until your body understands it. You look so graceful!

To travel, you simply repeat these actions, now to the left. You've taken one step forward with your left foot onto its toes. Your left palm is gripping your left thigh; your right palm is above your head. Begin to rotate your arms, the right arm down and forward, the left arm back and up, and remember to follow your left hand with your head, turning it to the left. At the same time, pivot on your left foot and turn your body to the left. Continue the arm rotations. When your left palm is above your head, simultaneously snap the palm so that it's facing left, the fingers pointing forward at about a 45-degree angle, snap your face forward, and turn your body forward. Also at the same time, take a small step forward with your right foot onto its toes as you plant your left foot flat, transfer-

ring the weight and power to the left leg. As you take that step, place your right palm on your right thigh, thumb on the outside of the thigh, fingers on the inner thigh.

Now you can keep going forward, alternating left foot, right foot. Try it. Remember to maintain the bended-knees crouch throughout. Don't rise out of the crouch and go back down into it when you take your steps. Remember that as one foot steps forward onto its toes, you plant the back foot flat, to carry all the weight and power. And, of course, be mindful of fully extending your body, keeping your back straight, shoulders square, head and chin up.

Practice this traveling Xu Bu until you're executing it with full coordination of your legs, arms, body, and head.

Fantastic!

(continued)

HOLLOW STANCE (cont.)

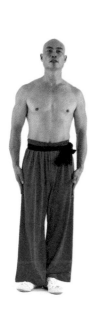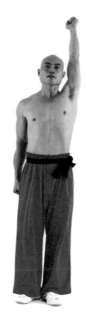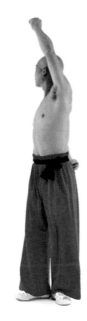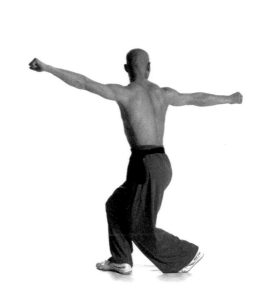

Now practice Xu Bu using your fists instead of palms.
Every other action is exactly the same.

Stand straight and relaxed, fully extended.

Lift your left arm straight up above your head, palm
forward, fist pointing to the sky, and place your right arm
straight down to your side, fist pointing to the ground.
Your arms are in the 6 o'clock position, with your left
hand pointing to the 12 and your right hand pointing to
the 6.

As you begin to rotate your arms, the left arm forward and
down, the right arm back and up, you follow your right
arm with your head, turning it to the right. Simultaneously, bend your knees and turn your body to the right,
pivoting on your right foot. Do not take a step; just pivot.
Execute all of these actions together so that you begin
rotating your arms, turning your body and head, and
bending your knees all in harmony.

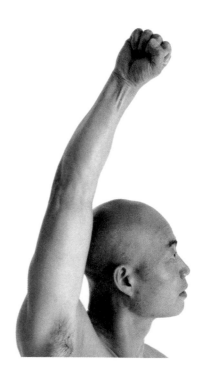

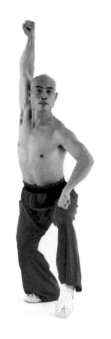
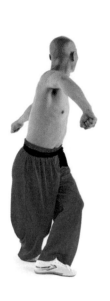
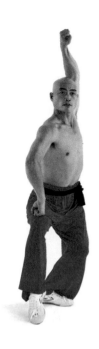

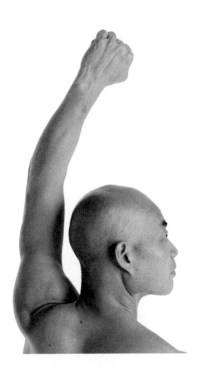

Continue rotating your arms. When your right fist is above your head, snap it so that your thumb is forward and your fist is pointing forward at about a 45-degree angle. Another way to say this is to point the "eye" of the fist—the center around which your fingers are curled—toward the ground. In Chinese, the eye of the fist is called *quan yan*. Be sure not to bend your wrist either backward or forward. Keep a very slight bend in that elbow—don't overextend it. At the same time, snap your head and turn your body to face forward, pivoting on the right foot. Also at the same time, take a small step forward with the left foot onto its toes. As you take that step, place your left fist on your upper thigh, with the thumb facing your hip and your knuckles facing in. Complete all these actions simultaneously and in full harmony.

Understand? Now you can continue to travel the fists version of Xu Bu precisely the same way you traveled the palms version. Practice this now. Awesome!

Meditation

You can't break bricks with just your mind or just your hand.

In the Shaolin Workout, you're developing the strength that comes from the harmony of physical, mental, and spiritual discipline. Please understand that your physical, mental, and spiritual powers are all one and the same. There is no separation of internal and external power. There is no difference between internal and external power. They are one and inseparable, like the body and the head. It is through expressing this harmony that a Chan Quan master like Sifu can break a stack of bricks with his bare hands, his head, his foot, his elbow.

People don't always understand this harmony. Some people cultivate the power of the mind, but they have no physical strength. Others build up their bodies, but their minds are weak and lazy. Both are incorrect. If your body is lazy and weak, it robs your mind of energy. If your body is strong but your mind is lazy, you lack the mental discipline and focus to train harder and push your body farther.

You cannot break bricks with just your mind alone. But at the same time, if your mind is not disciplined, you'll never believe you can break those bricks—and you won't, no matter how physically strong you are. You can break the bricks only when your body, mind, and spirit are in complete harmony.

As you go through your day today, be mindful of these harmonies. Express these harmonies of your body, mind, and spirit in your whole life.

"AMITUOFO! AMITUOFO! AMITUOFO!"

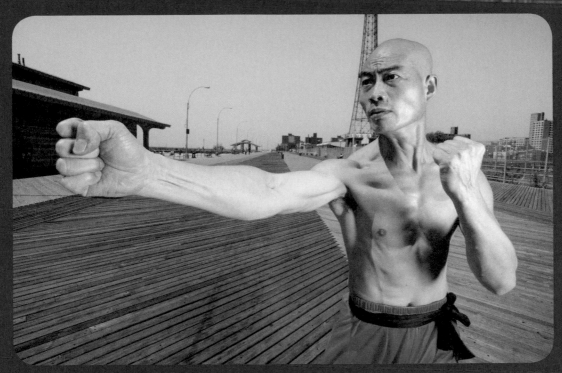

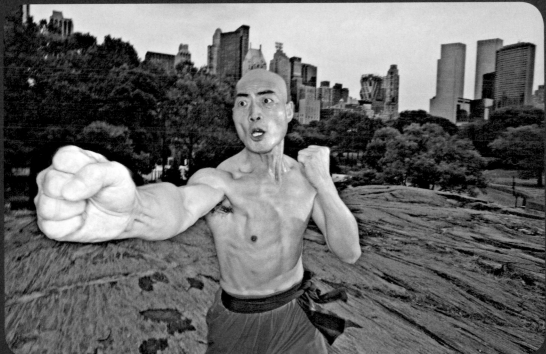

Review

"AMITUOFO!"
"AMITUOFO!"
"AMITUOFO!"

Congratulations! You've completed three-fourths of the program. As you go through your entire routine today, stretch a little farther, execute your kicks and strikes with more speed and chi. Keep working on perfecting all of your Shaolin Workout training.

Think back to your first few days. Feel how much more relaxed, more flexible, and stronger your body is today than it was when you started this program. You can bend farther, stand taller, sit straighter, walk faster. You're beginning to understand yourself better, to develop a warrior's confidence and calm, to apply the warrior's physical, mental, and spiritual harmonies and make your whole life better.

And you've only been training for 3 weeks. Think about how fantastic you're going to feel and look 3 weeks from now—and 3 months, and 3 years. You're so beautiful, and you're expressing it better than ever before. Keep going, and keep growing. Believe in yourself. Trust yourself. Have confidence in yourself.

"AMITUOFO!"
"AMITUOFO!"
"AMITUOFO!"

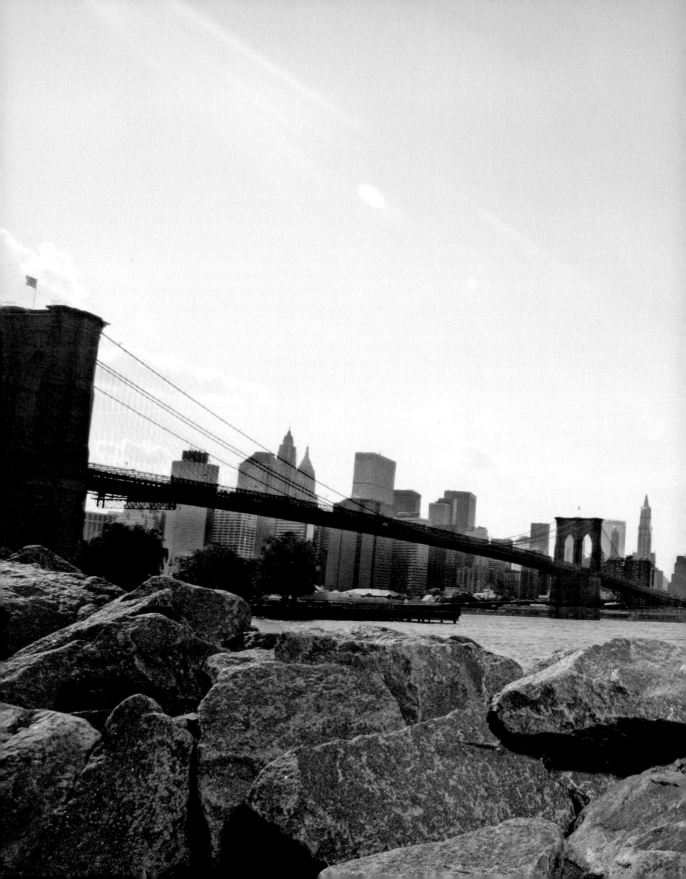

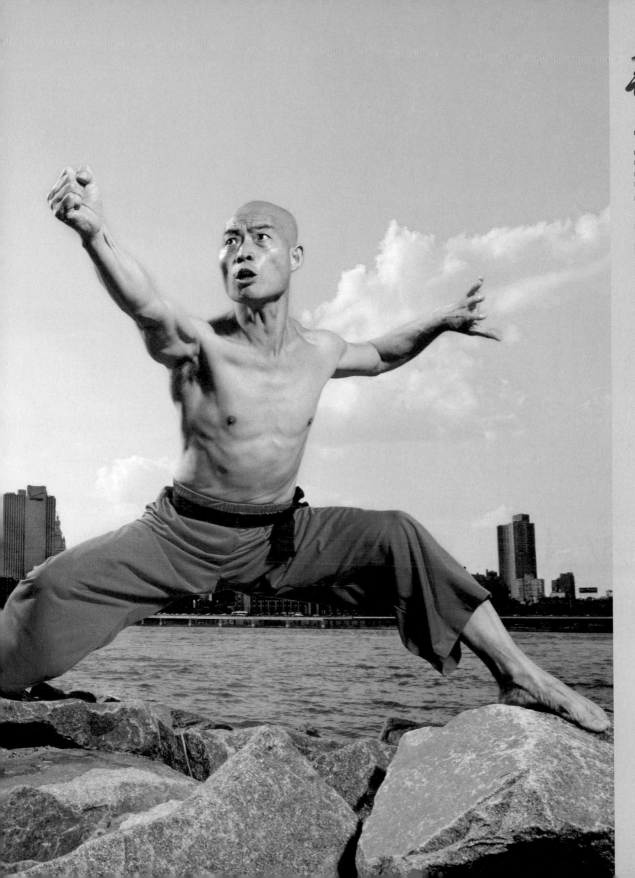

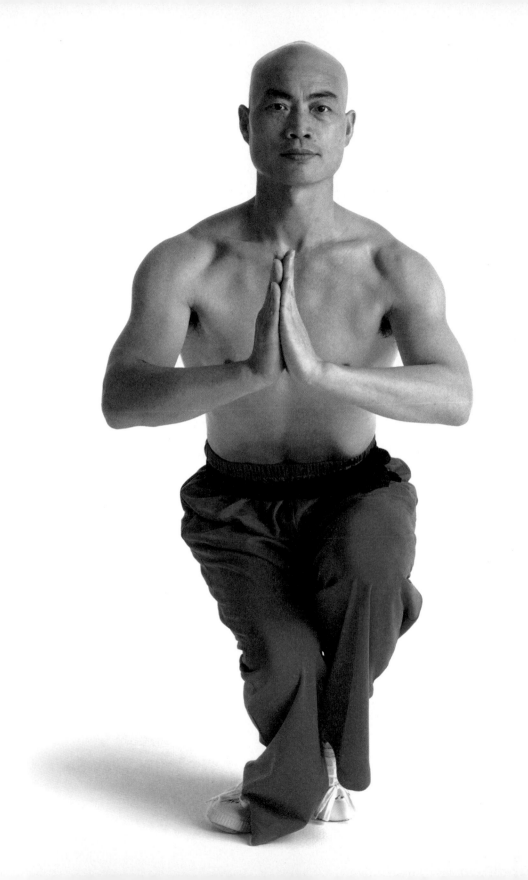

Front Snap Kick
T-Shaped Stance

"AMITUOFO!"
"AMITUOFO!"
"AMITUOFO!"

Begin with your daily routine. Today learn both a new kick and a new stance.

FRONT SNAP KICK
(Zhengtantui)

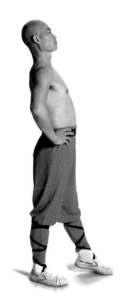 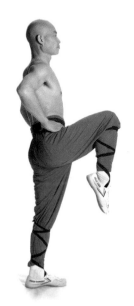 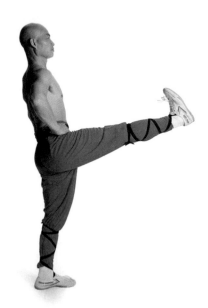

Zhengtantui (pronounced *jung-tan-twee*) is a snapping kick, like a spring. It is a style of kick different from those you've learned so far, because you bend your knee when you execute it. It incorporates both palm strikes and fist punches. Let's break it down into its parts, starting with the legs.

Learn the basic mechanics of the kick first. Support yourself with one hand against a wall, or holding on to a porch railing, the back of a chair, or a tree. For this example, kick with the right leg first. Lift your right thigh in front of you as high and as quickly as you comfortably can with the knee bent, your raised leg angled in front of your left leg, toes pointing down. All your weight is on your left leg.

Now flex your foot as you kick your heel straight up in front of you; then point your toes for landing and touch down on your toes, leg fully extended and knee locked. Fully extend your legs and body when your toes touch the ground.

Flexing your foot makes Zhengtantui much more of a workout than if you performed the kick with your toes pointed. Try kicking both ways, and you'll immediately feel the difference in your buttocks, hips, thighs, hamstrings, and calves when you kick properly, with your foot flexed.

Try it several times with the right leg; then switch and try it with the left.

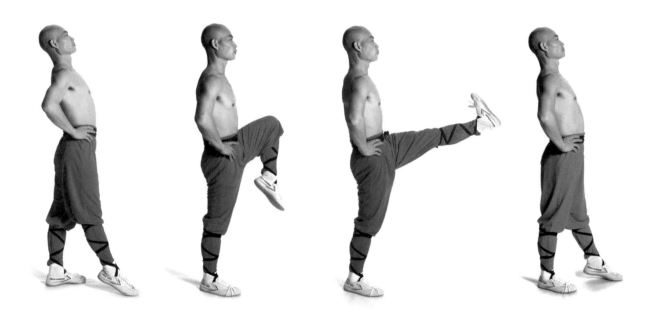

Now learn to travel, without a wall or other support. Learn it first without using your arms. Place your hands on your hips for balance. Stand straight and relaxed, fully extended; then take a small step forward with one foot—let's make it the left—onto its toes, your knee locked. Now, in one smooth move, lift your right thigh as high as you comfortably can, with the knee bent and your raised leg angled in front of your left leg, toes pointing down. All your weight is on your left leg.

Now flex your foot at the same time as you kick your heel straight up in front of you; then point your toes for landing and touch down on your toes.

Pause for a second; then go into a left flex kick: As you plant your right foot flat, transferring all the weight and power to that leg, lift your left thigh as high as you comfortably can with your knee bent. Kick your heel straight up with your foot flexed; then point your toes and come down on your toes, light as a feather.

Now you can do a right kick again. And so on.

Practice until you can march across the ground, flex-kicking left, then right, then left, and so on. Remember that each time you kick, your back leg is straight, knee locked, and that foot is flat on the ground. Remember to keep your body fully extended as usual, back straight, shoulders square, chin up, eyes on your beautiful future.

Fabulous!

(continued)

FRONT SNAP KICK (cont.)

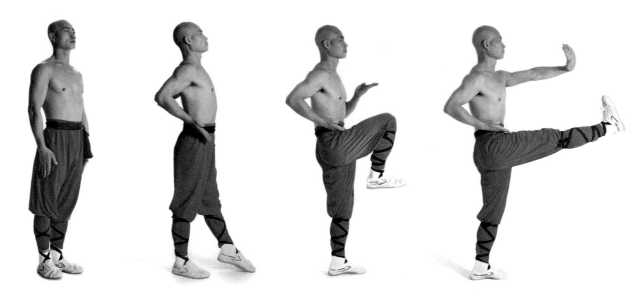

Now add the arms and strikes. Zhengtantui can be executed using both palm strikes and fist punches. Learn the palm strikes first. The palm strikes can be done in two versions. Here's how.

Stand straight and relaxed, fully extended.

Yu bei! Take a small step forward with the left foot onto its toes, knee locked, and at the same time chamber your palms, palms up, fingers pointed forward.

Zou! Plant your left foot flat as you lift the right thigh in front of you as quickly and as high as you can, with the knee bent. Now kick your heel straight up, foot flexed, and at the same time execute a palm strike with your left palm. Execute the right kick and left strike simultaneously and in harmony—pow! Don't lean forward. Keep your upper body fully extended, shoulders straight, chin up.

Practice this kick strike until you understand it. You're doing great.

Now travel, alternating kicks and strikes. You've kicked with your right foot and struck with your left palm. Now, as your right foot comes down onto its toes, leave your left arm out, and hold it there as you plant your right foot flat and lift your left thigh as high and as quickly in front of you as you can, knee bent. Kick your heel straight up, foot flexed, and simultaneously strike with your right palm as you slide your left palm back to your waist. Your arms should be like pistons, one snapping out to strike as the other snaps back to your waist.

Now keep traveling. Leave your right arm out and your left palm chambered as you plant your left foot flat and lift your right thigh. Kick with the right foot flexed, and simultaneously strike with the left palm as you chamber your right palm back at your waist. And so on, alternating kick strikes as you march forward.

Practice this now. Remember, you kick with your *right* foot and strike with your *left* palm and then kick with your *left* foot and strike with your *right* palm and so on, alternating.

Got it? Splendid.

Now practice Zhengtantui with another version of palm strikes. For this example, start with a right kick and a simultaneous left palm strike. Now, as you plant your right foot flat and lift your left leg, turn your palm so it is

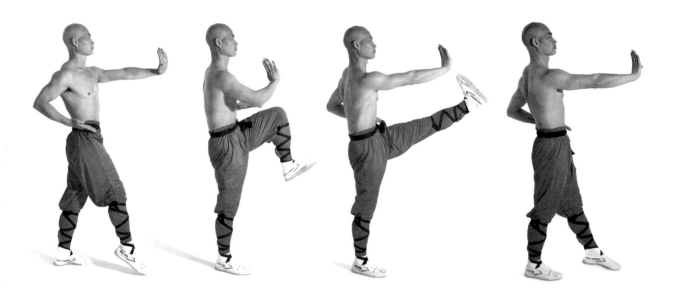

facing you and so the tips of your fingers are pointing right at a 90-degree angle, just as you've been practicing since Session 10. When you begin to kick up with the left heel, quickly lift your right palm behind the left and slide the left back to your waist so that your right palm strikes at exactly the same instant that your left foot kicks. Bam!

To travel, you just continue these moves, alternating left and right. Try it now, and repeat it until your body understands. You look fantastic!

Now learn Zhengtantui using fist punches instead of palm strikes.

Stand straight and relaxed, fully extended.

Yu bei! Take a small step forward with the left foot onto its toes, knee locked, and at the same time chamber your fists at your waist.

Zou! Plant your left foot flat as you lift the right thigh in front of you as quickly and as high as you can, with the knee bent and the toes pointed down. Now kick your right heel up, foot flexed, and at the same time execute a punch

with your left fist. Extend your arm straight out from your shoulder when you punch, and remember to twist your arm like a screw going into a wall as your fist comes up and punches—pow! Execute the kick and punch simultaneously and in harmony. Don't lean forward when you punch. Keep your body fully extended, shoulders straight, chin up.

Practice this kick punch until you get it.

To travel, just alternate kicks and punches. You've kicked with your right foot and punched with your left fist. Now, as your right foot comes down onto its toes, leave your left arm out as you plant your right foot flat and lift your left thigh in front of you. Kick your left heel up, foot flexed, and simultaneously punch with your right fist as you slide your left fist back to your waist. Your right arm twists out at the same time that your left arm twists back. Bam!

Now alternate feet and fists, marching toward the dolphins. Practice this until you've got it. Awesome!

That's Zhengtantui. Now learn a new stance today, Ding Bu.

T-SHAPED STANCE (cont.)

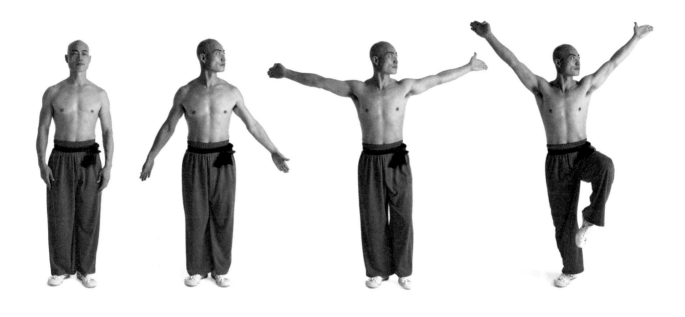

Stand straight and relaxed, fully extended. Lift your arms out at your sides and over your head, bring the palms together, and lower your arms in front of you. Remember to follow your left hand with your head. As you lift your arms, lift one thigh—for this example it should be the left—in front of you with the knee bent, angling your foot in front of your right lower leg, toes pointed down. Now bring the left foot down on its toes against the middle of the instep of your right foot. Do this as you lower your arms in front of you until your hands are in front of your middle Dentien.

There should be no weight on the left foot—all your weight is on your right leg. Make sure that you have your left foot fully extended and are up on its toes, not on the ball of your foot, and that your feet are touching.

Now slowly bend both knees and lower yourself into a crouch as low as you can comfortably go. Don't go all the way down so that your knees touch the ground. Remember to keep your body fully extended and your back straight. Don't curl your back or lean forward. Don't

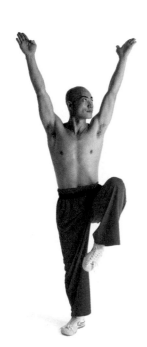 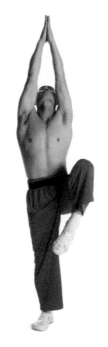 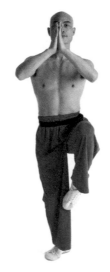 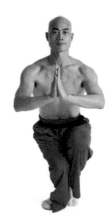

stick your butt out behind you. Keep your left foot fully extended and up on its toes. Keep all your weight on your right leg. Hold your lowest comfortable position for a moment; then stand up and lower your hands to your sides.

Pause for a moment. Now repeat, switching legs. Lift your arms above your head, bring the palms together, and lower your arms in front of you. This time, follow your right hand with your head. As you lift your arms, lift your right thigh in front of you with the knee bent,

angling your foot in front of your lower left leg, toes pointed down. Now bring the right foot down on its toes up against the middle of the instep of your right foot. Slowly bend both knees and lower yourself into a crouch as low as you can comfortably go. Hold it for a moment; then stand up and lower your hands to your sides.

Magnificent! That's all there is to Ding Bu. Keep at it until you can alternate feet as one graceful, fluid series of movements.

Meditation

Tiger head, snake tail.

In China, they have a saying, *"Hu tou she wei"* (虎頭蛇尾)—"Tiger head, snake tail." The tiger has a ferocious head, but his tail is as limp as a snake. That's a way of saying that we often start out a project with lots of energy, but we lose enthusiasm as we progress, and give up before we get the job done. You may know this from your own Shaolin Workout training. For instance, you may find yourself kicking high and quickly when you execute your first few Lihetui kicks, but by the fourth or fifth kick, you're feeling exhausted. Your form gets sloppy; your legs go limp as a snake. Your last few kicks have no power at all, no chi.

When you're training, the point when you begin to tire out is exactly the point when you should pour more chi into your routine. Focus all your energy on your next kick, and even more on the next, and more still on the next. Your last kick should be higher, stronger, and faster than your first.

Obviously, you can apply this principle to your entire life. Whatever task or project you're engaged in—starting a new diet, quitting cigarettes, taking evening courses in a new language, training to run in your company's charity marathon, or even healing a marriage or relationship that has hit a rocky patch—don't make excuses for giving up along the way. Remember, if you start making excuses, you'll never finish. Use your physical, mental, and spiritual harmonies to put more and more chi into it until you finish the race, get the job done, get your marriage right again. When the going gets tough, train harder. Whatever you're doing, finish stronger than you began.

"AMITUOFO! AMITUOFO! AMITUOFO!"

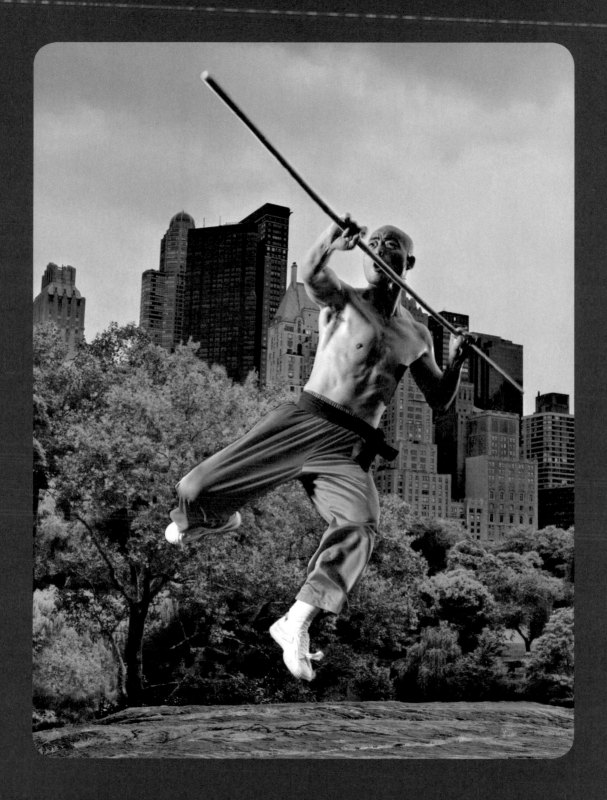

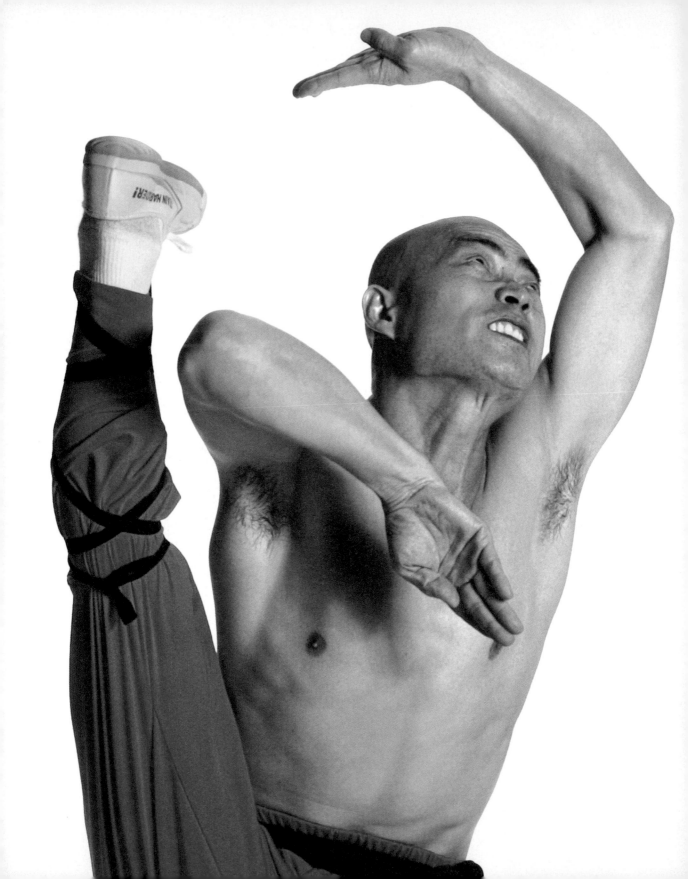

Side Flex Kick

"AMITUOFO!"

"AMITUOFO!"

"AMITUOFO!"

Execute your entire routine, up through practicing your Ding Bu. You're getting quite a workout now, aren't you? Feels great, doesn't it? You look amazing, too.

SIDE FLEX KICK
(Cetitui)

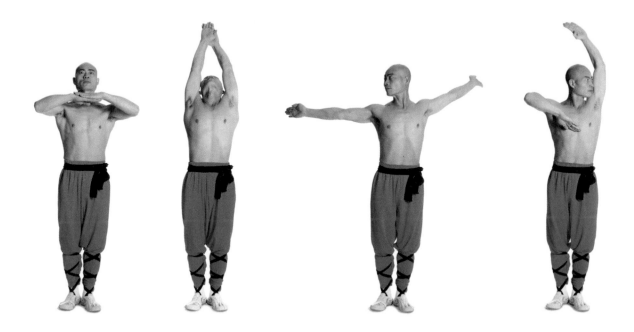

Cetitui (pronounced *seh-tee-twee*) is a flexed-foot kick straight out to the side. It incorporates your legs, arms, and head. Learn it in stages, beginning with just the arms.

For this example, learn the arm movements for a right kick first. Stand straight and relaxed, fully extended, feet together.

Quickly lift your arms from the center in front of you and slap your palms together in front of your chin. Remember not to swing your arms out to your sides and back in as you lift them.

Then lift them straight overhead, palms forward, and bring your palms together so that the fingers of one hand overlie the fingers of the other.

Now quickly lower your arms to a position where your *right* arm (which will be the kicking side) is straight out

to the side from your shoulder, palm forward and fingers pointed, and your *left* arm is also out to the side, but slightly higher than shoulder height.

Practice this as a set of three quick moves: *Yi*—slap palms in front of your chin. *Er*—lift arms straight overhead. *San*—swiftly lower arms. Keep your body and chest fully extended.

Add head snaps. You begin facing forward, chin up. Look up as you extend your arms overhead. Then, when you lower your arms, snap your head first to the left and then to the right, completing the head snap to the right at the exact moment that you complete the arm movement—ka-pow!

Quickly bend your arms, bringing your right palm up and in toward your chest, like the motion of a windshield wiper, and bending your left arm above your head. Snap

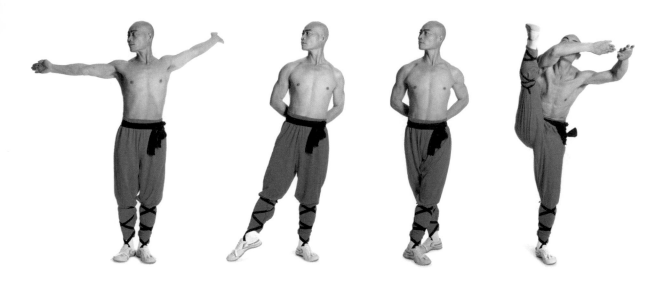

both arms at the same time—snap! And then, without a pause, snap them back out to the original position, fully extending your arms and body. Pow-pow!

Add a head snap. You're looking to the right when you begin. As you bend your arms, snap your head to the left, and as your arms snap back out, snap your head back to the right. Snap your head left-right in total harmony with your arms bending in and out—pow-pow!

Practice this arms-and-head sequence until you can do it quickly and in total harmony. Fantastic!

Practice the kick, first without the arms. Stand straight and relaxed, fully extended. Take a small step to the right with your right foot onto its toes, knee locked, without moving the left foot at all. Your right knee and foot should be pointing straight out to the right side when your toes touch down. This leg is "hollow," with all the weight on

your left leg. Keep your upper body straight, shoulders back, chin up. Don't lean to the right or the left.

Plant your right foot flat as you take a step to the right with your *left* foot. Plant your left foot past your right, with your left heel in front of your right toes and your left toes pointing 45 degrees to the left.

From this position, kick straight out to the right side with your right leg, knee locked, foot flexed. Kick as high and fast as you comfortably can; then point your toes for landing, and extend your body and arms up. Lower your foot onto its toes. Kick down as quickly as you kicked up; then land soft as a feather.

Practice this step to the right and right flex kick until you've got it.

Great!

(continued)

SIDE FLEX KICK (cont.)

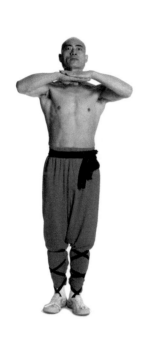 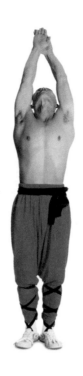 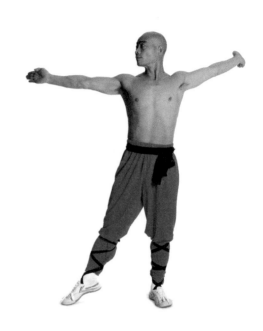

Now combine the arms, head, and legs into one harmony. Stand straight and relaxed, fully extended. Slap your palms together in front of your chin, lift your arms above your head, and quickly lower them, following them with your head as you look up and snap your head left-right. At the same time, take a small step to the right with your right foot onto its toes, knee locked. Your arms, head, and leg complete their movements at exactly the same instant and in complete harmony.

Now, holding your arms still and keeping your face to the right, plant your right foot flat and step past it to the right with your left foot. Flex-kick to the right with your right leg as you bend your arms in and back out and while you snap your head left-right. At the height of the

kick, point your toes for landing, and extend your body and arms; then bring your right foot down gently onto its toes. Your arms, head, and leg move in total harmony, beginning and ending at precisely the same instant— ka-pow! Remember to keep both knees locked, with your weight on your back leg, and fully extend your body to the sky. Don't lean your body in toward or away from the kick.

Understand? Practice it slowly at first, just getting all the elements down; then add more speed and chi with each repetition.

Practice kicking to the left, simply reversing the direction of your movements. Slap your palms together

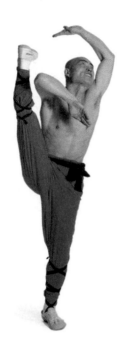

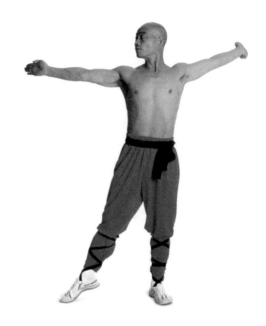

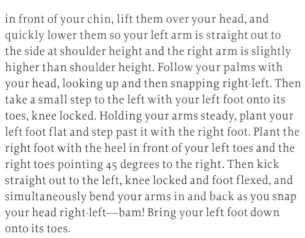

in front of your chin, lift them over your head, and quickly lower them so your left arm is straight out to the side at shoulder height and the right arm is slightly higher than shoulder height. Follow your palms with your head, looking up and then snapping right-left. Then take a small step to the left with your left foot onto its toes, knee locked. Holding your arms steady, plant your left foot flat and step past it with the right foot. Plant the right foot with the heel in front of your left toes and the right toes pointing 45 degrees to the right. Then kick straight out to the left, knee locked and foot flexed, and simultaneously bend your arms in and back as you snap your head right-left—bam! Bring your left foot down onto its toes.

Practice these left kicks until you've got them down. Then practice alternating right and left until you're repeating them with speed and chi.

Outstanding!

If you want to train harder, there's another version of Cetitui you can practice when you feel you've gotten the first version. In this version, don't step *past* your forward foot with your back foot. Take a smaller step with your back foot and kick. Then step and kick again. And again. You'll find that because you're taking smaller steps, you kick more often. More chi! Train harder!

Meditation

The person who has $10 wants $100. The person who has $10 million wants $100 million.

In the modern world, we are surrounded by things we think we want. We want those celebrity-endorsed sneakers. We want a wider-screen TV. We want a bigger house. We want a fancier car. We want a Rolex. We want that new cell phone with the extra function our almost-new cell phone doesn't have.

We want all these things because we think they will make us happier. But acquiring these things is not the same as achieving happiness. No matter how much wider your TV screen gets, it's still the same old you sitting there staring at it. No matter how fancy and prestigious your new Lexus is, somebody else is going to pass you in a Jaguar that's fancier and more prestigious. The person who has $10 wants $100. The person who has $10 million wants $100 million. As long as you equate acquiring things with achieving happiness, you'll never be happy. It's a treadmill, never ending.

True happiness comes from a life that is fulfilled, not just filled up with things. It's not bad to acquire those things, but it is bad if you let wanting them and chasing after them distract you from your real goals and true happiness. You'll never enjoy your life that way. The truly happy life is a life of action, not distraction. True happiness comes from mastering and polishing your life. It comes from self-respect and self-confidence and from developing harmony and balance so that you can savor *this* moment, here and now, for the beautiful gift it is. Happiness is spreading peace and love to the people around you. That's the warrior's way.

"AMITUOFO! AMITUOFO! AMITUOFO!"

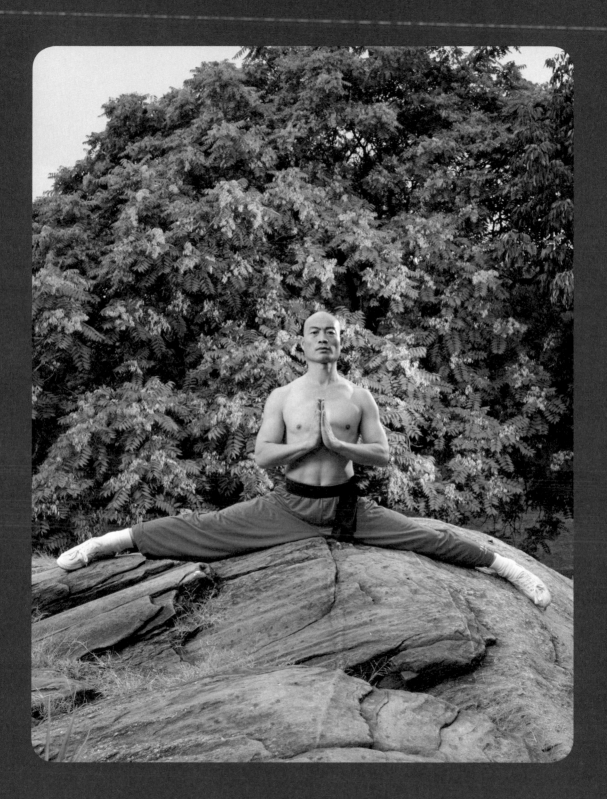

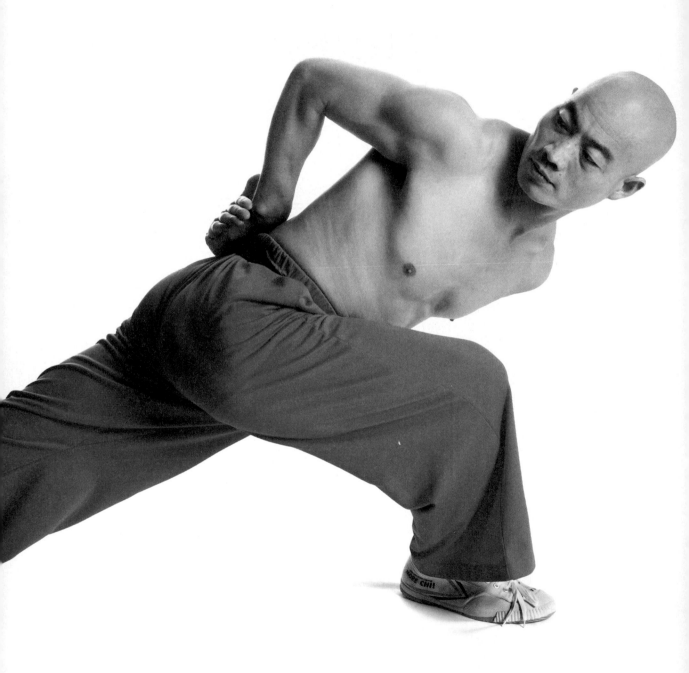

SESSION 24

Crossed Stance

"AMITUOFO!"
"AMITUOFO!"
"AMITUOFO!"

Go through your entire routine, putting more chi into every move.
Kick higher! Punch faster! More chi! Train harder!

CROSSED STANCE
(Tsa Bu)

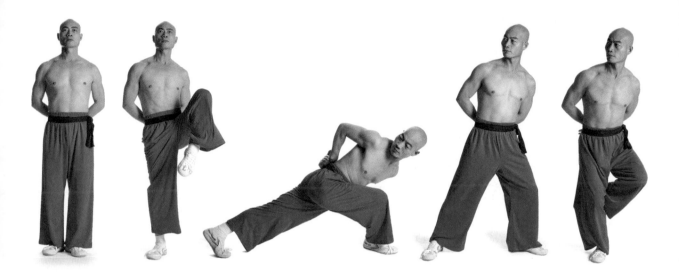

Tsa Bu (pronounced *tsah boo*) combines arm rotations, palm strikes, steps, your body and head. Learn the legs first; then add the other elements.

For this example, begin with the left foot. Stand straight and relaxed, fully extended, feet together. Fold your arms behind you. Lift your left thigh as high as you comfortably can beside your right leg, toes pointing down. Step with the left leg behind your right leg and to the right as far as you comfortably can, pivoting slightly on your right foot. Bring the left foot down onto the ball of the foot; your heel should be in the air so that it's in line with your right foot, with the toes facing the middle of your right foot. Learn to step far enough with the left foot so that your right thigh is parallel to the ground. As you step to the right, lean your body to the left, keeping it fully extended with the chest facing forward, your right shoulder pointing up, your left shoulder pointing down.

When you complete this step, your body should be one straight line angling up from your left foot all the way up to your head. Don't curl your body, and don't overlean. Make a straight, angled line with your entire body.

Understand? Practice this step with the left leg until your body gets it. Then practice it to the right, simply reversing direction.

Excellent.

Now learn to travel.

For this example, begin with the left foot again. Stand straight and relaxed, fully extended, feet together. Fold your arms behind you. Step to the right with your left leg onto the ball of the foot, with the toes facing your right foot. As you take the step, remember to lean your

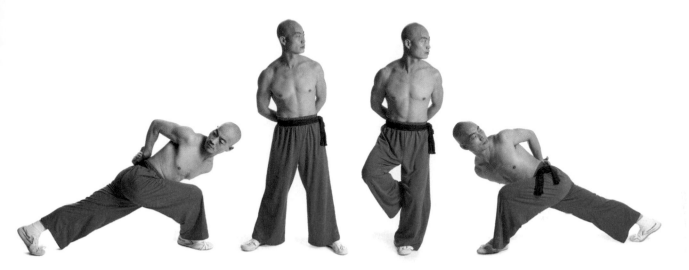

body to the left, keeping it fully extended, with your chest facing forward, right shoulder up, left shoulder down.

To travel to the right, step past your left foot with your right foot and plant it flat slightly more than shoulder width from the left foot, toes forward. Then, as far as you comfortably can, step to the right again with your left foot, onto the ball of the foot, fully extended, toes facing the right foot.

You can keep traveling to the right this way, step-and-go, step-and-go, all the way to Miami and the dolphins. Practice this now until your body understands it.

Now learn to reverse direction and travel to the left. Begin as you've been practicing, stepping to the right with your left foot onto the ball of the foot and leaning your body to

the left. To travel to the left, step to the *left* with your *left* foot and plant it flat at shoulder width from the right foot, toes forward. Then lift your right thigh with the foot behind your left leg, pivot slightly on your left foot, and step to the left onto the ball of the foot, your right leg fully extended, the toes of your right foot pointing to the left foot. Keep your chest forward and lean to the right as you step, making a straight line angling up from the ground to your head, with your left shoulder pointing up, right shoulder down.

Now you can continue traveling to the left, step-and-go, step-and-go, all the way to Iceland and the polar bears.

Practice these traveling Tsa Bu steps to the right and to the left until you've got them down.

Beautiful.

(continued)

CROSSED STANCE (cont.)

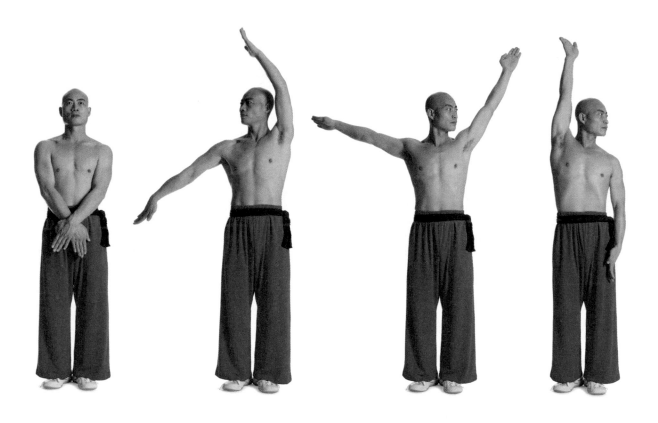

Now practice the arm rotation and palm strike, first without the feet. Stand straight and relaxed, feet together. The arm rotation is very similar to what you've been practicing in Xie Bu and Pu Bu. Start the Tsa Bu sequence with your wrists crossed over your groin and your palms flat in front of you. For this example, cross the *left* wrist over the right.

Rotate your arms counterclockwise, left arm leading up and to the left, right arm following.

Follow your left hand with your head, turning first to the right and then to the left. Continue the arm rotation and bring your forearms together in front of your navel, right arm on top of the left, right palm down, left palm up.

Chamber your left fist as you strike to your right side with your right palm, chopping straight out to your right side like a blade chopping the bad things out of your life, with the edge of your palm facing up and the

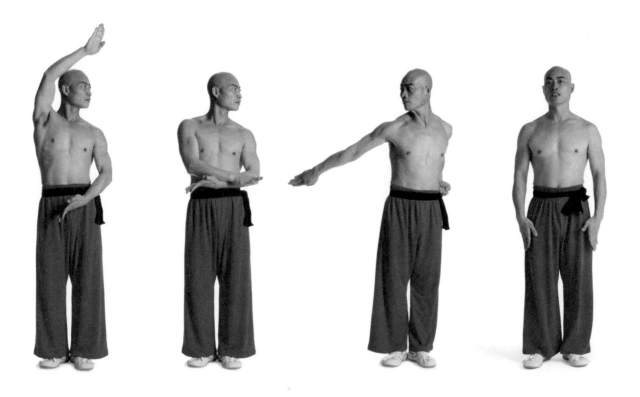

palm facing behind you. Your extended right arm should be positioned lower than shoulder height. In addition, it should be straight out to your side, not behind you. Remember to use the power of opposites when you strike, pulling your left shoulder back when you chamber your fist and throwing your chest open—pow! Also remember to snap your head to the right when you strike. And be mindful of fully extending your body and your arms.

To strike to the left, simply reverse. Begin with your right palm over your left at your groin. Rotate your arms clockwise, bring your arms together in front of your waist with the left over the right, and strike to your left side, chopping to the left with the blade of your left palm as you chamber your right fist and pull your right shoulder back to open your chest—bam! Remember to snap your head to the left when you strike. Understand? Good.

(continued)

CROSSED STANCE (cont.)

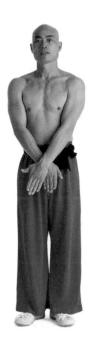 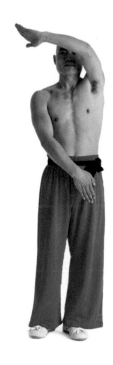 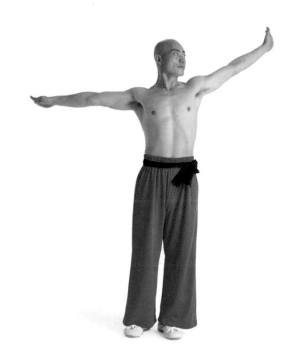

Now put the arm rotation, strikes, steps, and head turns altogether into one smooth movement, as shown above.

For this example, you're beginning with a strike to the right. Stand straight and relaxed, fully extended, feet together, with your wrists crossed over your groin, left on top of right.

Begin to rotate your arms counterclockwise, remembering to follow your left hand with your head. Rotate your arms to the 6 o'clock position, right arm above your head, left arm down at your side.

Bring your forearms together in front of your navel, lifting your left thigh beside your right leg.

Step to the right with your left leg fully extended onto the ball of the foot, toes facing your right foot, and at the exact same time, strike to the right. Chop the blade of your right palm straight out to the side as you chamber your left fist and pull your left shoulder back, throwing your chest open to give the strike extra chi—bam! Remember to lean your body to the left as you step and strike, keeping your chest forward, right shoulder up, left shoulder down, to make a straight line angling up from your left foot to your head. Don't twist or curl your body. Don't lean too far to

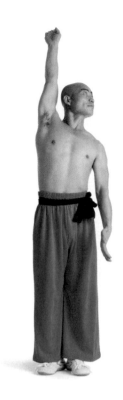
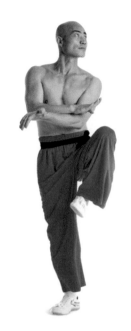
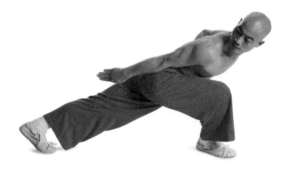

the left, and don't lean to the right—make a straight line. Also, remember to snap your head to the right as you strike. Execute the step, the strike, the lean, and the head snap simultaneously and in total harmony.

Practice this step and palm strike to the right until you're comfortable with it. Be mindful of fully extending your body at all times. You look awesome.

Now you can travel and keep striking to the right, like this.

Execute a right step and palm strike. Then cross your palms in front of you, left over right, and begin another counterclockwise arm rotation, and step to the right with your right foot. Your arms should come to the 6 o'clock position as you plant your right foot. As you bring your forearms together in front of your waist, lift your left thigh with the left foot *behind* the right leg, which makes it easier to travel quickly. Step to the right with the left foot onto the ball of your foot at the same time that you strike to the right and chamber your left fist—pow! Remember to snap your head to the right as you strike.

You can continue traveling right-palm strikes to the right, all the way to the dolphins.

(continued)

CROSSED STANCE (cont.)

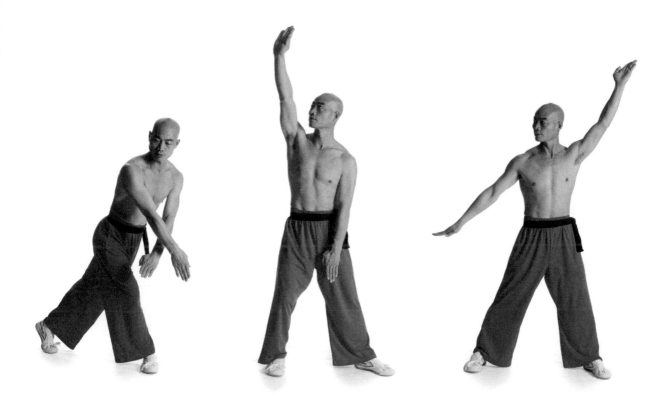

To travel and strike to the left, simply reverse direction. After you've executed a right step and right-palm strike, cross your wrists in front of you, right wrist over the left, and begin a *clockwise* arm rotation.

Step to the *left* with your left foot. Your arms should reach 6 o'clock at the same moment that you plant your left foot, toes forward.

Bring your forearms together in front of your waist, left on top of right, and at the same time lift your right

thigh, with the right foot behind the left leg. Step to the left with your right foot onto the ball of the foot at the same time that you strike to the left with the blade of your left palm, chambering your right fist and pulling your right shoulder back. Remember to lean to the right as you step and strike, keeping your chest forward. Remember to snap your head to the left when you strike. The step, strike, lean, and head snap happen simultaneously and in full harmony—bang!

Now you can continue stepping and striking to the left this way, all the way to the polar bears.

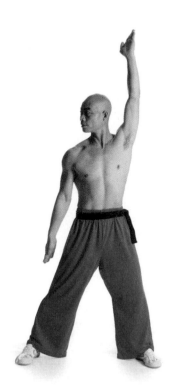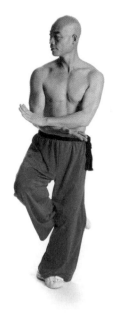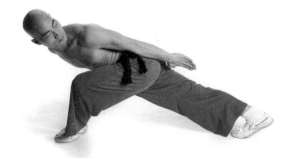

Practice traveling Tsa Bu to the right for a few steps; then reverse and travel to the left, and then to the right, until you can step and strike in either direction.

If you're training in a small space, you can alternate right and left Tsa Bu strikes without traveling. Simply strike to the right, and then reverse and strike to the left, and then reverse and strike to the right again.

Practice until you can execute it as one smooth, uninterrupted sequence of moves. Step and strike right; then immediately begin to rotate your arms and step and strike to the left; then instantly begin to rotate your arms and step and strike to the right again, and so on, left and right, left and right. Bam! Bam! Bam! Bam!

Fantastic! The dolphins are weeping, they're so jealous!

Meditation

Every action can be a form of action meditation.

When Da Mo saw the monks of Shaolin Temple sitting in no-action meditation for hours and hours every day, he realized that things were out of balance. They were exercising their minds, but their bodies were growing stiff and weak. And the more uncomfortable their bodies became, the less they were able to focus their minds and properly meditate.

So, with the help of former generals Hui Guang and Seng Chou, Da Mo introduced the monks to action meditation. To do that, he created the four most important sutras in Shaolin Temple's history. Some people believe that sutras are lessons, or preachings, that can be expressed in words alone. But just as there is action and no-action meditation, there are action and no-action sutras. There's no difference between action meditation and no-action meditation as methods of cleansing and polishing the mind. The four sutras Da Mo created are action sutras: Wu Xing Quan (five animal forms); Luohan Shi Ba Shou (18 Luohan palms); Yi Jin Jing (muscle- and tendon-changing sutra); and Xi Sui Jing (bone-marrow-washing sutra).

In our modern world, few of us have time to sit still and meditate for hours. This is where action meditation comes in. And you don't need to be practicing your kung fu kicks and stances to practice action meditation. Every action of your day can be a form of meditation. Washing the car, walking to the bus stop, vacuuming a rug, giving the dog a bath, folding laundry, typing a report, brushing your teeth. Play some ball with your kids. Climb a tree like a monkey. Make dinner. Make love. There are unlimited ways to meditate. You simply bring to each action the same focus and discipline you bring to your kung fu kicks and strikes. Whatever action you're engaged in, be fully mindful of the moment, relaxed in your mind and body, conducting yourself with a warrior's focus and confidence, no matter how trivial or mundane the action might seem. No moment in your life is trivial. Every moment is a gift. Every second of your day is an opportunity to continue polishing your life.

Whatever you do today, try doing it as an act of meditation. Extend your body, and extend your mind.

"AMITUOFO! AMITUOFO! AMITUOFO!"

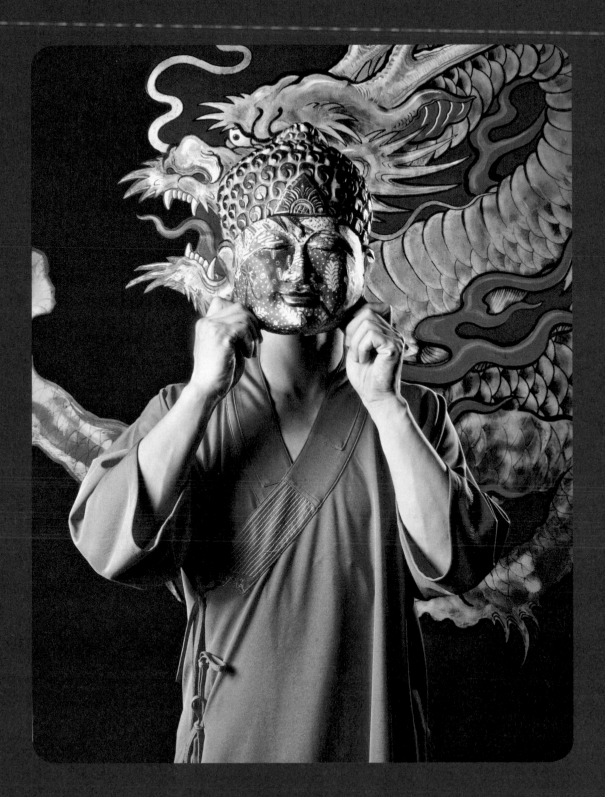

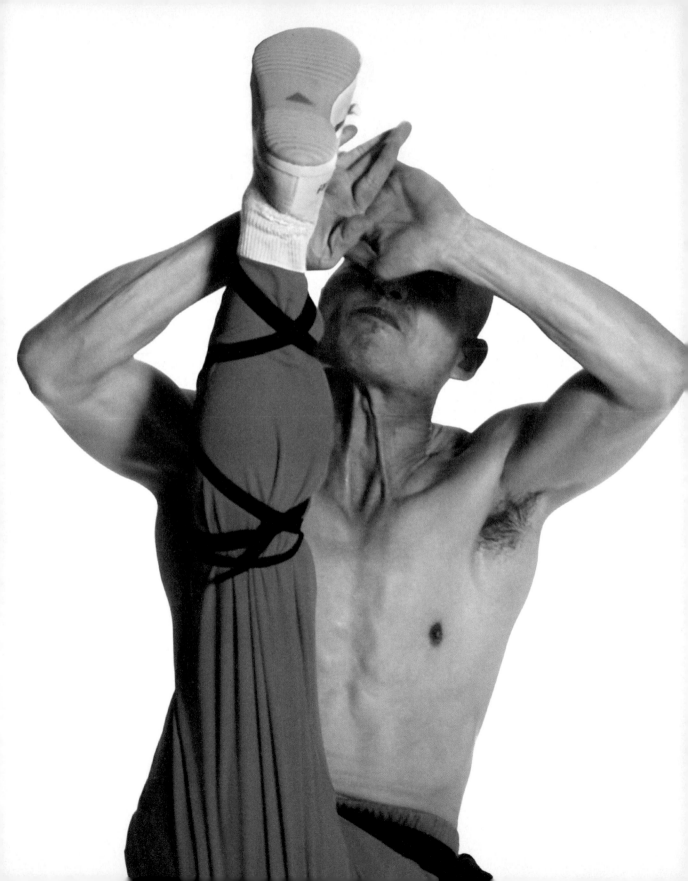

SESSION 25

Outside Crescent Kick

"AMITUOFO!"
"AMITUOFO!"
"AMITUOFO!"

Begin with your regular training. Faster! Higher! Challenge yourself.

OUTSIDE CRESCENT KICK
(Waibaitui)

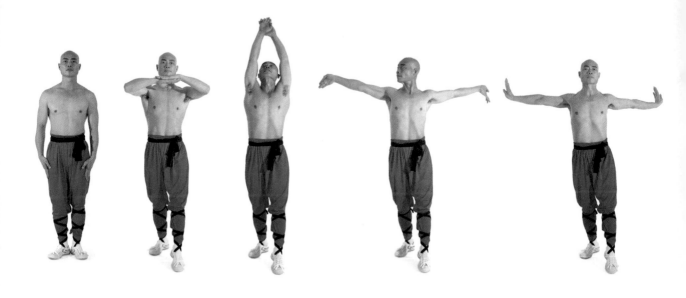

Waibaitui (pronounced *wy-by-twee*) is a kick that makes an arc from the center out and back to the center, with palm slaps. Learn the kicks first; then you'll add the palm slaps.

Stand straight and relaxed, feet together, fully extended. For this example, begin with a right kick. Just as you do in Zhengtitui and Lihetui, lift your arms from the center in front of you and slap your palms together in front of your chin as you take a small step forward with your left foot onto its toes, knee locked.

Quickly lift your arms straight above your head, palms crossed and facing forward.

Quickly bring your arms down to shoulder height and a little behind you, fully opening your chest, at the same time that you snap your palms downward. Follow your right palm with your head, snapping your head to the right.

Now snap your palms up and facing out to the sides, simultaneously snapping your face forward. Hold your arms in this position as you practice doing your kicks.

Now, just as you've been practicing with Zhengtitui, plant your left foot flat and kick your right leg straight up in front of you, knee locked and right foot flexed. When your

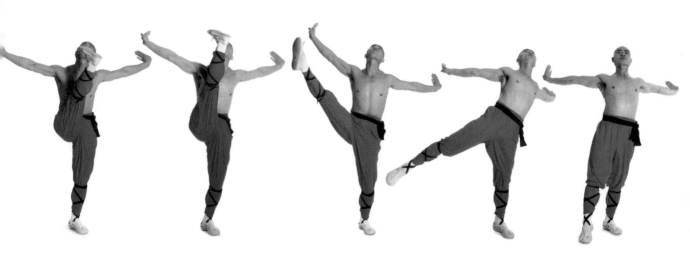

foot comes closest to your head, express an explosion of chi—pow!

Point your toes and fully extend your whole body from your toes to your head—and both arms, too! Continue to kick your leg out to the right in a circle as high as you can reach and as wide and as far back as you comfortably can; then continue back to the center, touching your toes down in front of you at their original position.

Don't forget to keep your left foot planted firmly and keep both knees locked. Don't lean into the kick, or bend or twist your body. Keep your body straight and

your eyes forward, and extend your whole body up to the sky.

Practice this right kick several times. You'll feel it working your whole body, from your head, shoulders, and chest down through your back, hips, and buttocks, and all the way down your legs to your toes.

When your body understands the right kick, practice kicking with your left leg. Then practice alternating them right and left, increasing your height, speed, and chi with every kick.

Beautiful!

(continued)

OUTSIDE CRESCENT KICK (cont.)

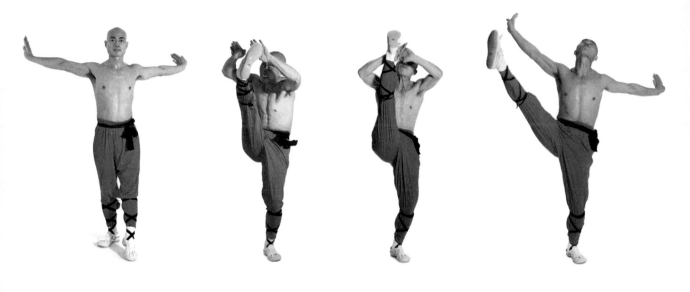

Now add the palm slaps.

As you begin your kick, your arms are at shoulder height and slightly back. Quickly bring them in front of you as you kick, with your palms together side by side, thumbs touching, fingers pointing straight ahead.

Slap your foot at the height of the kick—the instant you express an explosion of chi—then quickly bring your arms back out to shoulder height as you lower your foot onto its toes. Fully extend your body, throwing your arms wide and your chest open, with your head up. Fully extend both legs. Don't lean into the kick or bend your knees.

If you can't reach your foot with your palms, practice slapping your thighs to start with. Also, you can practice at first without lifting your arms out to your sides. Put

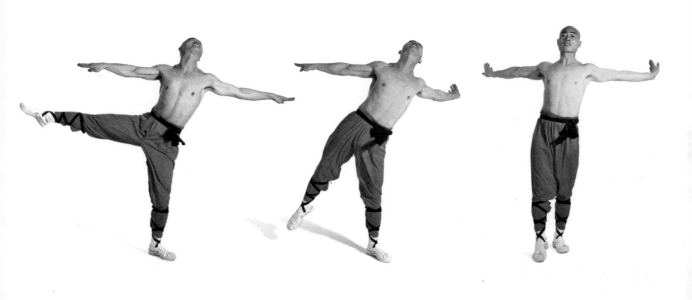

your palms together, thumbs touching and palms down, and hold them up off your right shoulder. As you kick with the right leg, slide your palms in, slap your right thigh, and continue sliding your palms over to your left thigh as your right foot touches down on its toes. Kick up with the left leg, sliding your palms in to slap your thigh; then continue to slide your palms over to your right thigh as your left foot touches down on its toes. And so on.

Keep practicing, and you will eventually master this kick. Extend a little farther with each kick that you practice, kick a little higher and faster, and you will get it. And the way it works your whole body—from your toes up through your hips and buttocks to your back, chest, shoulders, arms, and head—will feel great.

Meditation

Chi can be used positively or negatively.

Chi is the life force that connects all things. Trees and flowers have chi. Insects and amoebas have chi. Inanimate objects have chi. Chi flows through the entire universe.

Chi is the force you channel and use every time you do your Shaolin Workout training. Like an electric current or nuclear power, chi is an extremely powerful force, but it is neither positive nor negative in itself. However, we can put it to positive or negative use. When you get angry, you can literally feel the chi being used negatively—your face gets hot, and you feel the chi like an electrical current in your trembling fingers. You can hear the chi's negative use in your voice as it trembles and gets louder or higher.

When you do your training, you can feel the chi flowing positively through your limbs. Your whole body heats up with chi. At the U.S.A. Shaolin Temple, if you walk in while a class is in session and a few dozen students are training together, the chi literally hits you like a blast of heat from an oven.

Through your training, you're learning to put your chi to use in a positive way, directing it to polish your mind and body and life, to sculpt your life into a beautiful work of art. By developing your physical, mental, and spiritual harmonies, by learning how to flatten your heart and remain calm and relaxed at all times, you're learning how *not* to express your chi in negative, angry, hurtful, frustrating ways.

As you go through your day, remind yourself to stay loose and relaxed, letting that positive chi flow through you and connect you to those around you, spreading peace and love, not anger or hurt.

"AMITUOFO! AMITUOFO! AMITUOFO!"

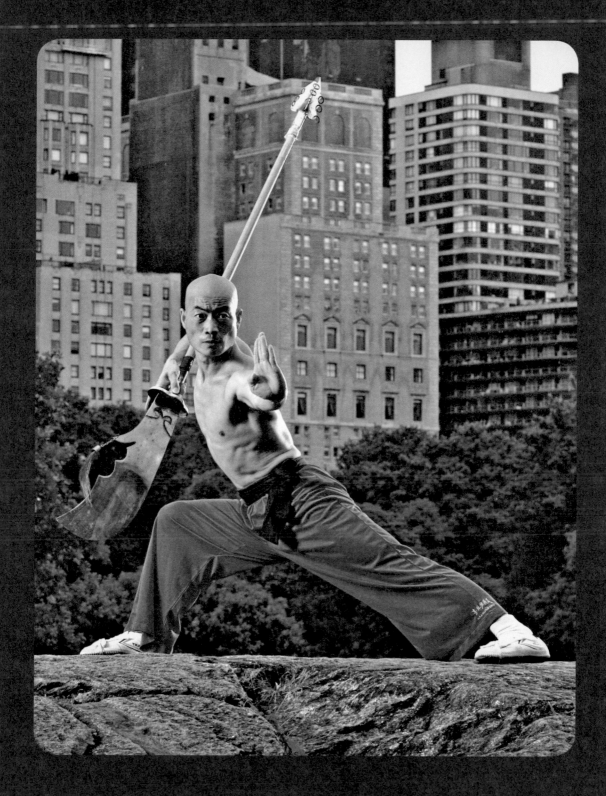

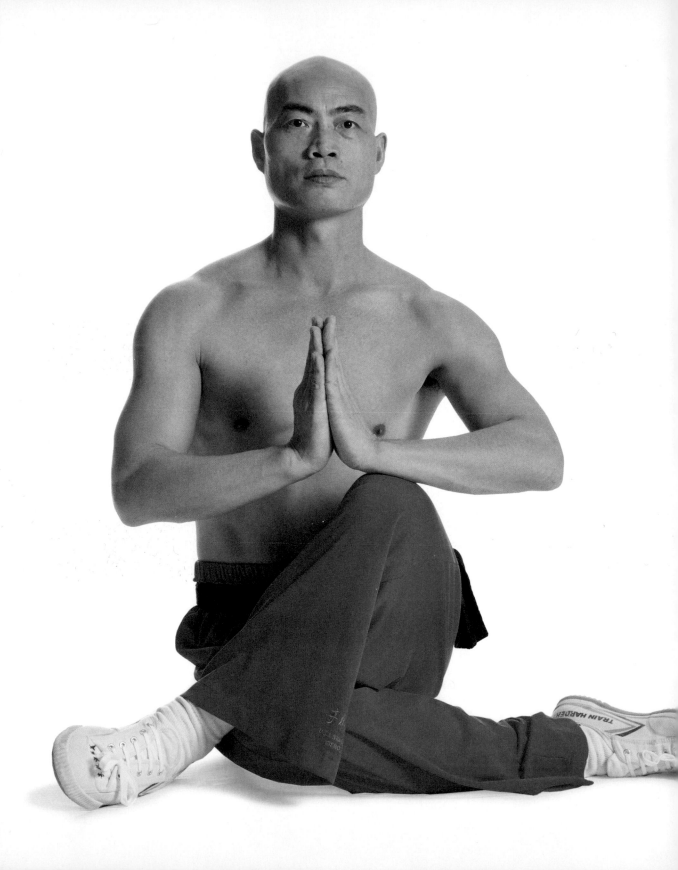

Crossed Seated Stance

"AMITUOFO!"
"AMITUOFO!"
"AMITUOFO!"

Do your daily training, all the way from your wrist rotations
through your Waibaitui kicks, perfecting and polishing every part of your
Shaolin Workout. Then learn a new stance.

CROSSED SEATED STANCE
(Zuopan)

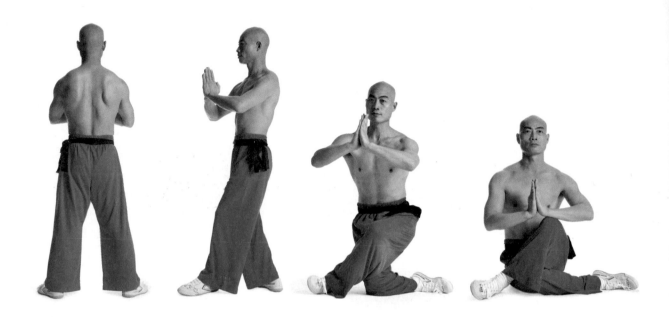

Zuopan (pronounced *zoh-pan*) is an excellent stance for developing your coordination and balance. Learn it slowly and gently at first; then build up speed and chi as you master it.

Learn the legs first, with your palms together in a praying gesture in front of you.

Stand straight and relaxed, fully extended, feet planted firmly, slightly farther apart than shoulder width so your legs make a strong inverted-V shape.

Now turn your body to the left, pivoting on both feet; don't lift your feet or take a step. As you turn with your feet in one place, your legs will naturally go into a crossed stance, with your right knee behind your left knee.

When you've turned 180 degrees, so that you're now facing the opposite direction of where you started, go down slowly into a cross-legged crouch. Go down gently until you're sitting on the ground, with your legs crossed, the left leg over the right thigh. Be mindful of keeping your body fully extended, your back straight, head and chin up.

To return to your original standing position, you simply "unwind" yourself. As you begin to rise

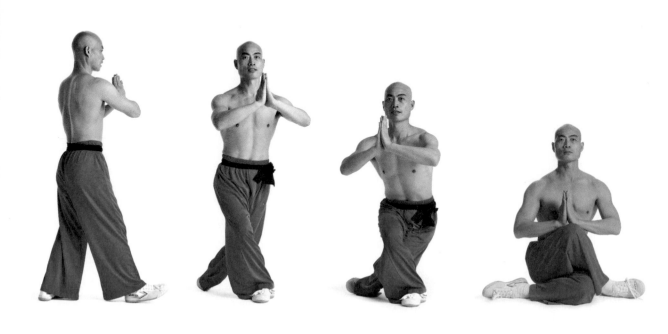

from the ground, turn your body to the right, pivoting on both feet. Keep turning and pivoting until you're standing in your original position. Remember not to lift your feet or take a step. Just pivot in one spot.

Understand? Practice it a few times. Go slowly and gently at first. Don't come crashing down to the ground. Gradually increase speed as you master the turns.

Now learn to execute Zuopan in both directions, alternating left and right turns. Execute a turn and crossed-leg crouch to the left; then rise and turn to the right until you're standing in your original position. Now turn and pivot to the right, coming around 180 degrees, and lower yourself gently into another crossed-legged crouch on the ground, with your right knee over your left thigh. Then rise and turn to the left, back to your original position.

Now you can keep alternating left and right turns, twisting up and down like a screw turning into and out of the ground.

Magnificent!

(continued)

CROSSED SEATED STANCE (cont.)

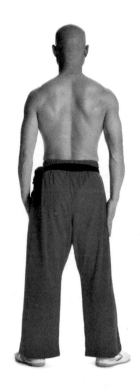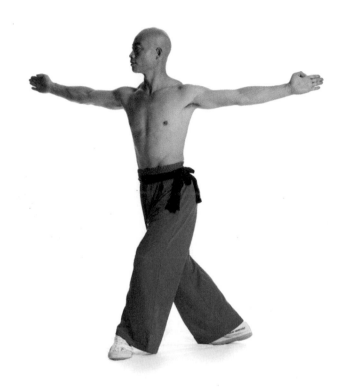

Now add the arms to this stance. Start the sequence with your hands down at your sides. Begin to turn your body to the left, pivoting on both feet while you lift and extend your arms at your sides. As you complete the turn and begin to lower your body toward the ground, bring your palms together in front of your middle Dentien in the praying gesture.

Now just hold your hands in the praying gesture as you rise and turn to the right, back to your original position. Then pivot 180 degrees to the right and descend into another crossed-legged crouch, holding your hands in the praying gesture throughout. Then rise and turn back to the original stance. And so on, turning left and right, left and right.

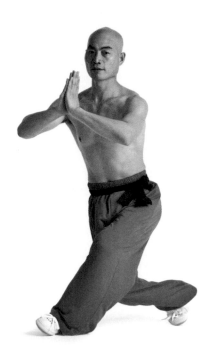

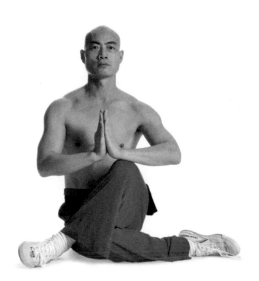

Practice this 10 times, alternating left and right turns.
Yi—left. *Er*—right. *San*—left. *Si*—right.... Remember to
keep your body fully erect, head up, at all times. Don't curl
or slump your back.

Got it? Gorgeous!

Meditation

Action becomes no-action. No-action becomes action.

People often ask how Shaolin monks reconcile kung fu action with the peaceful nature of Buddhism. It seems like a contradiction.

But in fact there is no contradiction. Both action and no-action are forms of meditation. Sifu says, "*Dong zhong sheng jing. Jing zhong sheng dong*" (動中生靜， 靜中生動). Action becomes no-action. No-action becomes action. Another way to say it is "*Dong chan bu dong chan*" (動禪不動禪).

The goal of meditating is to empty the mind of images and thoughts. To cleanse your mind and cleanse your heart. To be fresh and clean, a pure mind in a pure body, like a newborn.

There are unlimited ways to meditate. You will find for yourself the best way for you to meditate. It may be climbing a tree or a mountain, or swimming or playing tennis. Whatever helps you cleanse your mind and your heart is your way of meditating.

A lot of Buddhist monks and masters—in fact, most instructors—teach only sedentary meditation. Their students believe that sitting in the lotus position is the only way to meditate. But that's only one way to meditate. If you want to sit and meditate, you don't have to sit with your legs crossed in the lotus position—especially if you find that uncomfortable. How can you cleanse your mind if your knees and back are aching? You can sit and meditate with your legs stretched out, or any other way that's comfortable and helps you to cleanse your mind. There are no rules. Find the best way for yourself to live your beautiful life.

That's why Sifu teaches action meditation. If you're uncomfortable sitting for hours in silence, get up! Say something! Life is for living. Life is exercise. Life is action. Do some action meditation. Think of Da Mo's bone-marrow-washing sutra: Sweat the terrible things out from inside you; then take a shower and rinse them off and down the drain! Now your body and your mind are so fresh and so clean!

Action becomes no-action. No-action becomes action. The action is the philosophy and the philosophy is the action. In Buddhism there are many thousands of sutras, and no sutra. When you practice the martial arts, there are many styles, and no style. In Chan Buddhism, Chan means everything and nothing. Keep it simple. The simple way is the beautiful way. Don't confuse yourself. Understand yourself. Create your own destiny, and your own way to express your beautiful life.

"AMITUOFO! AMITUOFO! AMITUOFO!"

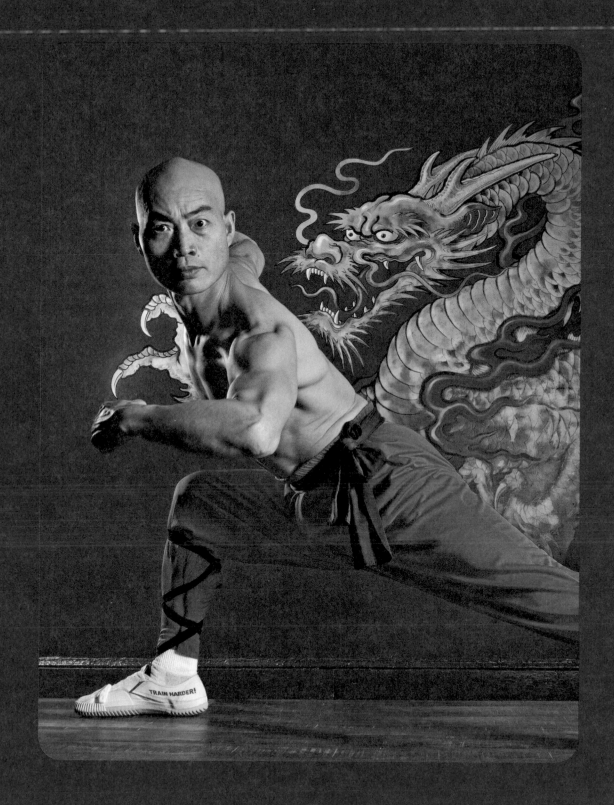

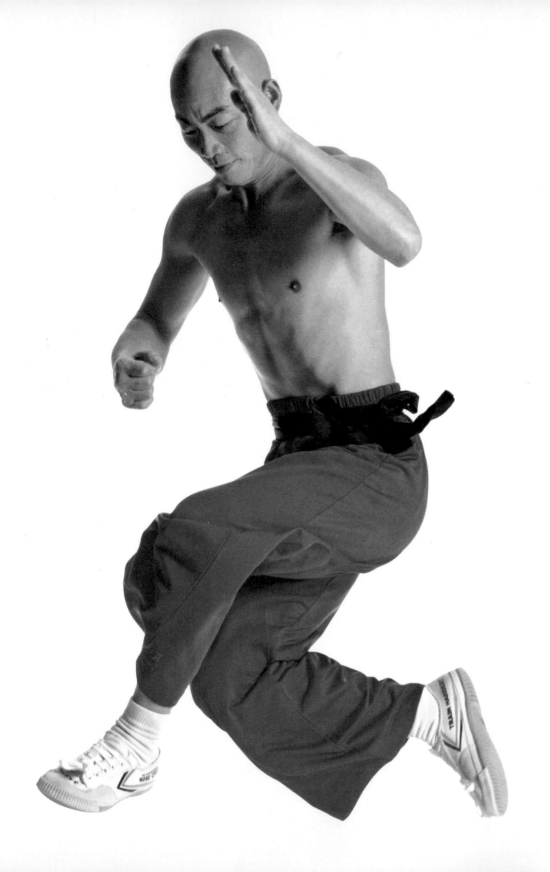

SESSION 27
Luohan Sleeping

"AMITUOFO!"
"AMITUOFO!"
"AMITUOFO!"

Execute your entire daily routine.

Stretch a little farther today than you did yesterday. Kick a little higher, faster, and stronger. Execute all your movements more fluidly. Polish your movements, and polish your life. Look at yourself—how different you look and feel from when you started. You look magnificent. More chi! Train harder!

LUOHAN SLEEPING
(Luohan Shui Jiao)

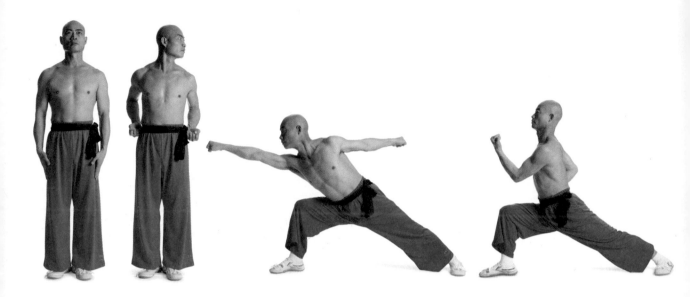

Eighteen Luohans guard the Shaolin Temple, and all of Buddhism. You often see statues of them in temples. Each Luohan has his own name and character—this one is fierce and menacing, another is laughing, and so on.

Since this is the last movement you'll learn in the Shaolin Workout, let's go out with a bang. Luohan Shui Jiao (pronounced *lo-han shwee jow*) incorporates a little bit of almost everything you've been practicing in your workout: a stance, a kick, palms and fists, an arm rotation, a hop, and a crossed-leg descent to the ground. That may sound like a lot, but you're ready for it, and as you practice it, you'll see how each element flows naturally into the next to make one beautiful and powerful sequence. You'll love the feeling of accomplishment you get when you master it.

Learn it in stages; then you'll connect them into one fluid form.

Stand straight and relaxed, fully extended, feet together, arms at your sides.

Yu bei! Quickly chamber your fists and snap your head to your left.

Zou! Step with your right leg to the right side into a Gong Bu stance, with your left leg fully extended. As you step, lean your body to the right, making a straight line angling from your left foot to your left hip to your left shoulder to your head. Popping up your left hip helps you make this neat line. You should make such a neat line that someone could lay a broom

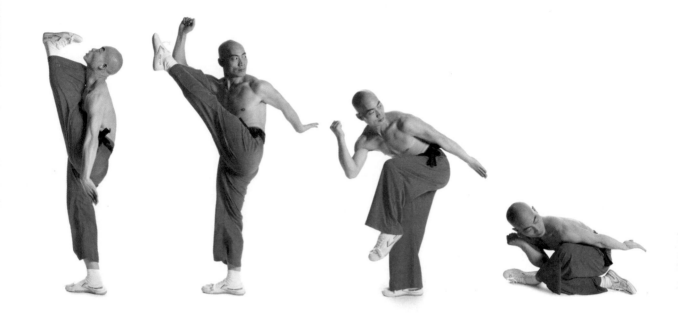

against your left side. Be mindful of fully extending yourself.

Also as you step and lean, extend your arms straight out from your shoulders and parallel to the ground, right arm over right leg and left arm over left leg. This position is called Dan Bien Shin (單鞭式). It's like you're holding two presents in your fists at the ends of your fully extended arms—one for Christmas and one for New Year's. When you extend your arms, follow your right fist with your head and look straight along your right arm and out past your fist to see the dolphins.

Maintaining the Gong Bu stance, pivot your left foot and turn your body to the right. At the same time, punch forward and up with your left fist, like a boxer punching

an uppercut, so that your left fist strikes up in front of your chest, with the back of your hand facing forward. Also at the exact same time, twist your right arm back to chamber your fist. Bam!

Now you will execute a kick, a palm strike, and arm rotations. Keeping your right foot planted firmly, execute a Zhengtitui kick with your left leg, knee locked, foot flexed. At the same time that you kick with your left leg, open your left fist into a palm and chop straight down like a blade cutting the bad things out of your life.

When your left foot comes closest to your head, point your toes, pop your whole body even higher, and begin to rotate your arms. Your left arm continues to rotate back and up, and your right arm rotates forward and down.

(continued)

LUOHAN SLEEPING (cont.)

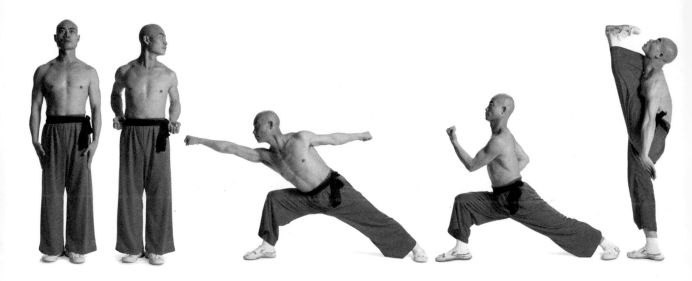

Make a full rotation with your left arm and rotate it behind you, palm facing up, as though you've just pulled a blanket up over yourself. Meanwhile, when your right arm has rotated in a circle forward and down to where your fist is by your waist, bend your right elbow and strike with your fist up to your right ear—like you're grabbing a pillow and dragging it to your head.

As you complete the kick, plant your left foot flat in front of your right foot so that your legs are crossed, left leg in front of the right.

Quickly lower yourself into a crossed seated crouch on the ground. Don't land with a bump—touch down as soft as cotton. Complete your arm rotations at the same time as you complete your descent to the ground. As you reach the ground, lean your body to the right. You look like Luohan

sleeping on the ground, with a pillow (your right arm) under his head and a blanket over himself to keep warm. Think of the times you've fallen asleep and left the air conditioner on and then woken up cold and with stiff joints. Stay warm! Just like you should stay warm in your heart!

Practice all of the preceding movements until you can do them fluidly.

Got it? Excellent. Now add the final element, a hop-jump.

Perform all of the preceding movements as instructed, but this time, as you are kicking down with your left leg and beginning your arm rotations, hop off your right foot so that for a second your entire body is in the air. Plant your left foot flat in front of you, and plant your right foot to the left so that your legs are crossed, left leg in front of the right.

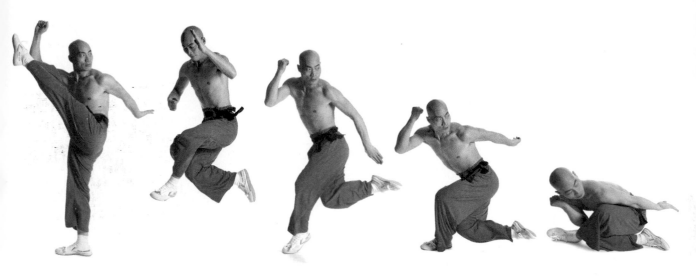

Quickly lower yourself into the crossed seated crouch on the ground, completing your arm rotations at the same time that you complete your descent.

Yes, those are a lot of separate elements to put together into one move, but you're ready for them at this point in your Shaolin Workout. As you practice Luohan Sleeping, be mindful of the elements that you execute simultaneously and in full harmony:

- When you take the Gong Bu step, you simultaneously extend your arms straight out from your shoulders to the Dan Bien Shin position.
- When you begin the Zhengtitui kick with your left leg, you simultaneously chop down with your left palm.

- When your left leg reaches the height of the kick, you pop your body and begin to rotate your arms.
- As your left leg descends, you hop up off the right foot, continuing the arm rotations.
- When you bring your feet down with the legs crossed, you lower your body into a cross-legged crouch, completing it at the exact same time that you complete the arm rotations.

As you practice Luohan Sleeping, you'll understand how all those elements flow together into one fluid and powerful sequence. Keep practicing, and you will master it. You will enjoy ending your daily routine with this powerful sequence of moves.

Fantastic! Give yourself a hand. You've earned it.

Meditation

The true warrior uses the martial arts to spread peace and love.

Someone who doesn't understand the true meaning of kung fu might say, "Luohan Sleeping is a nice-looking move, but I don't see what use it would be to you in a fight. So why do you practice it?"

But you know better now. You know that learning kung fu is not learning how to beat people up. You know that the true value of learning kung fu is the calm, confidence, and respect you develop from being the master of your own body, mind, and life. The real goal of kung fu is to polish your body and mind, achieve harmony and balance in your life, and help others by your example to seek the same qualities. In that sense, it's no contradiction to say that the true kung fu warrior uses the martial arts to spread peace and love.

"AMITUOFO! AMITUOFO! AMITUOFO!"

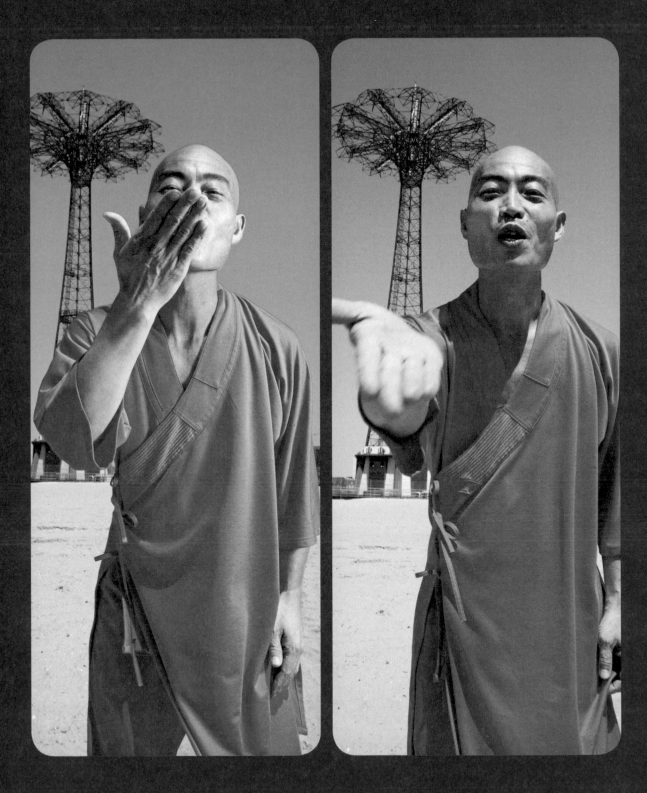

SESSION 28

Review

"AMITUOFO!"
"AMITUOFO!"
"AMITUOFO!"

It's graduation day! Today, review your entire Shaolin Workout in one smooth, powerful session, from wrist rotations through those once-difficult stretches, right on up through Xie Bu and Caijiao to Luohan Sleeping.

Stand in front of a mirror and look at yourself. You're so beautiful! Are you amazed at the way you've already transformed yourself in just 28 sessions? You should be. You *are* amazing.

No, you don't know "everything there is to know" about kung fu. That could take lifetimes. But you do now know the fundamentals on which much of kung fu is based. You've strengthened your body, made it more flexible, and improved your balance and coordination, all of which are crucial. If you choose now to go on studying kung fu, you'll be working from a solid foundation. If you choose not to learn more kung fu, regular training in the Shaolin Workout will help keep your body strong, trim, and graceful, while the confidence and self-respect will radiate out through your life.

Just as important as the kicks and stances, you've been introduced to the philosophy. You realize that kung fu is much more than just fancy moves. It is a warrior's way of mastering his body and his life, of understanding himself and others, of expressing his inner as well as his outer beauty, of finding balance and harmony in everything he does, of spreading calm and peace and love everywhere he goes.

Today, think about everything you've learned as you've progressed through the Shaolin Workout. Not just the stretches and movements but what you've discovered about yourself. Congratulate yourself. You really have begun a complete transformation. Promise yourself that you will continue the process and train regularly, whether it's through kung fu classes or on your own. Don't backslide. Yesterday is past. Today is beautiful. Tomorrow will be even more beautiful! Feel and see all that you've achieved. Maintain it, and keep going. Don't be afraid to grow. Trust yourself. Have faith in yourself. Train harder!

Apply what you've learned from the workout to your entire life. Put more chi into everything you do—your work and studies, your family and relationships, your hobbies and other activities. Your body, your mind, and your life are precious gifts. Don't waste them.

"AMITUOFO!"
"AMITUOFO!"
"AMITUOFO!"

3. Train Farther!

Now that you've completed the Shaolin Workout, it's quite likely you'll want to continue your kung fu training. You've learned the fundamentals. You've felt the wonderful transformation in your body and mind that comes from this training. You've sweated and maybe groaned and worked past the initial soreness. You've had such fun challenging yourself with a cool new move every day. You want more. And there's so much more to learn—not just about kung fu, which is a whole universe of styles and movements you've only just begun to explore, but about *yourself*, the infinite universe of your own being.

Sifu Shi Yan Ming strongly encourages you to continue to train, to learn, to grow, to transform. Unlimited knowledge should be your goal.

It may not be everyone's destiny to come to New York City to enjoy the life-changing experience of training with Sifu in person at the U.S.A. Shaolin Temple. But remember, you make your own destiny, and you must find your own way to keep training. (If you are planning a visit to New York, you can contact the temple in advance and arrange to join a class or take a private lesson. You can find all the information you need at the temple's Web site, www.usashaolintemple.org.)

Because of kung fu's enormous popularity, there are thousands of martial arts schools and classes around the world. Unless you live in a remote wilderness, a school or classes should be available nearby. You can find them easily online or in your local yellow pages.

Through the Shaolin Workout, you've had the unique opportunity of learning the pure essence of Shaolin Temple kung fu from the authentic and world-renowned master Sifu Shi Yan Ming. There are as many different styles and teaching methods out there as there are schools and teachers. Before choosing a school, observe a class. Try to meet the teacher or master before signing up. Does the school feel right? Does the teacher? Go with your instincts.

If you can't or don't want to train in a formal class setting, you should very definitely continue practicing your Shaolin Workout on your own. Sifu will write more books teaching you other movements. But be mindful that kung fu isn't all about adding more and more movements to your repertoire. You can spend your entire life and derive enormous satisfaction simply from polishing and perfecting the movements you've learned through *The Shaolin Workout*. Sifu says it takes only one move to tell whether or not someone has skills.

You've come so far in just 28 sessions. You've done such beautiful work transforming your body and your mind. Don't let it all go to waste. Commit yourself to training every single day. There should never be a day when you cop out by telling yourself you're too busy or too tired to train. Are you too busy or tired to eat? To go to the bathroom? Your training is no less important. Make the time. You've got the energy—the chi is in you. Just get up and start. In an instant you'll feel so good to have that chi flowing again that you'll breeze through your entire routine. You've learned how to do your training anywhere—in your bedroom, a hotel room, at (or on!) your desk, in the aisle of a plane. Don't give yourself any excuse for not training every day.

You've earned yourself a spectacular gift. Don't toss it away. Every day for the rest of your life, in everything you do, cheer yourself on. More chi! Train harder!

Amituofo!

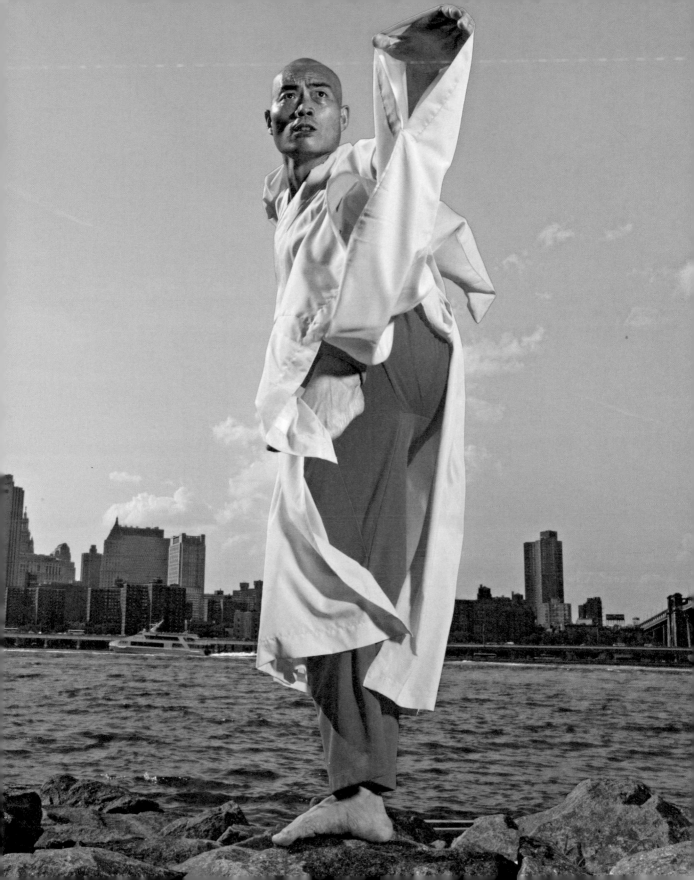

Index

Boldface page references indicate illustrations.

stationary version, 134–35, **134–35**
traveling version, 130–33, **130–33**
Breast Mountain, 10
Buddhism. *See also* Chan Buddhism
    creation of, 9
    Xiao Xing, 9

C

Caijiao (front slap kick), 139–43,
    140–43
Cetitui (side flex kick), 239–43, **240–43**
Chan Buddhism
    on enlightenment, 32–33
    founding of, 9, 11
    meditation on
        acquiring things, 244
        beauty, 82
        body as gift, 126
        Buddha inside yourself, 136
        celebration, 104
        change and richness of life, 190
        chi, 50, 264
        cleansing the mind, 272
        confidence, 182
        destiny, 170
        facing problems and challenges, 144
        finishing strong, 236
        flattening your heart, 116
        goal of kung fu, 280
        happiness, 244
        harmony, 76, 220
        laziness, 210
        life and body as art, 158
        paradise inside you, 170
        patience and perseverance, 92
        power, internal and external, 220
        practice, 68, 92
        relaxing mind and body, 58
        respect and love, 202
    role of monk in the world, 18–19

    rules, 24
    universal balance, 116
Chan Quan. *See also* Kung fu
    action meditation, 32
    animal forms, 11–12
    Da Mo and, 11
    speed as key, 95
    training, 3–5, 36
Chi
    in birds, 210
    harmony, 76
    positive and negative use of, 264
    power, 50, 264
Chi kung, 22
Chong Quan (fist punch), 124–25, **124–25**
Clothing, 34
Commitment, to training, 31–32
Confidence, 38, 82, 182, 244
Crescent kick, inside (Lihetui), 205–9,
    206–9
Crescent kick, outside (Waibaitui), 259–63,
    260–63
Crossed seated stance (Zuopan), 267–71,
    268–71
Crossed seated stretches, 112–15, **112–15**
Crossed stance (Tsa Bu), 247–55, **248–55**
Crouched stance (Pu Bu), 193–201, **194–201**

D

Da Mo
    action sutras, 256, 272
    Drum Mountain, 190
    founding of Chan Buddhism, 11
    meditation of, 10–11
Da Mo Ting, 10
Dan (confidence), 182
Dan Bien Shin position, 277
Dentien, 150–51
Desire, 9
Dharma, 9, 16

Luohan Shi Ba Shou (18 Luohan palms),
  256
Luohan sleeping (Luohan Shui Jiao), 275–80,
  276–79

M

Ma Bu (horse stance), 147–56, **148–57**
  one-step version, 154, **154–55**
  stationary version, 156, **156–57**
  traveling version, 148–52, **148–53**
Meditation
  action meditation, 11, 14, 32, 58, 256, 272
  no-action meditation, 58, 256, 272
  purpose of, 32
  topics
    acquiring things, 244
    beauty, 82
    body as gift, 126
    Buddha inside yourself, 136
    celebration, 104
    change and richness of life, 190
    chi, 50, 264
    cleansing the mind, 272
    confidence, 182
    destiny, 170
    facing problems and challenges,
      144
    finishing strong, 236
    flattening your heart, 116
    goal of kung fu, 280
    happiness, 244
    harmony, 76, 220
    laziness, 210
    life and body as art, 158
    paradise inside you, 170
    patience and perseverance, 92
    power, internal and external, 220
    practice, 68, 92
    relaxing mind and body, 58
    respect and love, 202

Muscle
  fast, long, 36
  slow, short, 35–36

N

Nail stance (Ding Bu), 232–35, **232–35**
Neck rotation, 54, **54**
Neck stretch, 54, **54**

O

Outside crescent kick (Waibaitui), 259–63,
  260–63

P

Palm strike
  in crossed stance (Tsa Bu), 250–55,
    250–55
  with front snap kick (Zhengtantui), 230–31,
    230–31
  pushing palm strike (Tui Zhang), 120–22,
    120–23
Paradise Buddhas, 2
Posture, 82
Power, 35–36
Prayer, 33
Pu Bu (crouched stance), 193–201, **194–201**
Pu Bu stretch, 102–3, **102–3**
Punch
  fist (Chong Quan), 124–25, **124–25**
  with front snap kick (Zhengtantui), 231
Pushing palm strike (Tui Zhang), 120–22,
  120–23

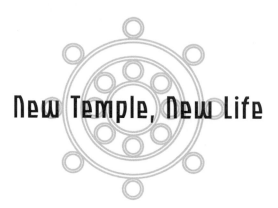

New Temple, New Life

Sifu Shi Yan Ming's goal is to build a replica of the original Shaolin Temple in China in upstate New York while maintaining a presence in Manhattan. The new temple will include the 72 chambers of authentic Shaolin training, where students and instructors can live and train winter, spring, summer, and fall.

In 2004 the U.S.A. Shaolin Temple launched the New Temple, New Life campaign devoted to raising funds to see this dream realized. The new temple will allow our community to grow by offering more classes, providing room and board, hosting summits and other special events, running corporate retreats and other team-building programs, and expanding our outreach to give more young people from economically disadvantaged backgrounds an opportunity to train.

Once the temple has room to grow, Sifu will be able to share his philosophy with anyone from around the world who is willing to train hard and learn. In this way, the temple will preserve the Shaolin legacy and spread its universal message: Strengthen your mind and body, understand yourself so that you can understand others, and help yourself so that you can help others. We ask all who desire to see the wisdom and compassion of 1,500 years of Shaolin tradition continued for this and future generations to contact us at the U.S.A. Shaolin Temple or at our Web site (www.usashaolintemple.org) to make a contribution.

Amituofo!

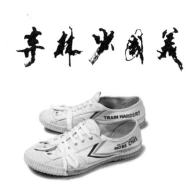